Wonderful Wheat
Hearty Grains for Healthy Homes

Enjoy Cooking
with Wheat.
and reading This
book. Anna Casbeer

Wonderful Wheat
Hearty Grains for Healthy Homes

By
Anne Casbeer

CFI
Springville, Utah

This is not an official publication of The Church of Jesus Christ of Latter-day Saints. The opinions and views expressed herein belong solely to the author and do not necessarily represent the opinions or views of Cedar Fort, Inc. Permission for the use of sources, graphics, and photos is also solely the responsibility of the author.

ISBN 13: 978-1-59955-173-9

Published by CFI, an imprint of Cedar Fort, Inc., 2373 W. 700 S., Springville, UT 84663
Distributed by Cedar Fort, Inc., www.cedarfort.com

LIBRARY OF CONGRESS CATALOGING-IN-PUBLICATION DATA
Casbeer, Anne.
  Wonderful Wheat: Hearty Grains for Healthy Homes / Anne Casbeer.
    p. cm.
  Includes index.
  ISBN 978-1-59955-173-9 (alk. paper)
  1. Cookery (Wheat) I. Title.

  TX809.W45C37 2008
  641.6'311--dc22

                    2008018888

Cover design by Jeremy Beal
Cover design © 2008 by Lyle Mortimer
Edited and typeset by Jessica Best

Printed in the United States of America

10 9 8 7 6 5 4 3 2 1

Printed on acid-free paper

Dedication

I need to thank my three boys for helping me evaluate each recipe as I tried the recipes on them first. Some became their favorite and some never worked (they aren't in this book). I would also like to thank those who have helped me to compile this book.

Table of Contents

Preface

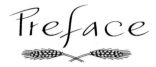

Wheat has been used throughout the ages for food, nutrition, and sustenance. It has been stored in times of plenty for times of famine. I collected and developed these recipes during those times of plenty. I was working and studying in research and development as a registered dietitian in the home and in a hospital. When my job outside the home and my marriage ended, I had three young children to care for. Being a single parent with little income, I soon entered the times of famine and used these recipes.

Wheat is an inexpensive source of protein and vitamins. It was an excellent way for me to give my family nutritious meals on a limited budget. I also collected and developed mixes to save money. I didn't have to buy fast-food or convenience foods. The mixes gave me the convenience of the quick meals and quick mixes for quicker meal preparations.

I'm always interested in developing recipes. Knowing the value of wheat in storage and in nutrition, I became interested in studying it. Being divorced with three young children to take care of, I had an even greater desire to learn of inexpensive but nutritious ways to feed my young family. I used my skills as a research dietitian to develop and compile recipes of wheat that my family would like.

Soon I started a bakery in my home, and I had 10 employees. We baked about 300 dozen goods (breads and cakes) a day, five days a week. We delivered daily to stores with a different route each day. Items not sold were then put into a freezer, and many customers came to the bakery to buy day-old items. I also made specialty cakes for weddings, birthdays, and other special occasions.

I later I experimented and developed wheat recipes at home. My recipes on wheat were overflowing. As a result I compiled this cookbook with most of our favorite recipes.

Notes and Tips about Wheat

Whole wheat berries are the full kernel that comes off the wheat staff in the field. They can be found in health food stores. One cup of whole wheat berries will yield about three cups when cooked. It is used in many recipes in this book.

If the cooked whole wheat berries are dried in the oven or a dehydrator, they are then bulgur. Bulgur can easily be made by cooking whole wheat berries either on the stovetop or in a slow cooker, much like rice. When cooked, it may puff and crack open but will be soft. Drain and rinse. Put on a cookie sheet and bake at 150 degrees, with oven door slightly open to let out the moisture. Another way is to use a dehydrator until thoroughly dry. Bulgur can be used whole or cracked. Cracked bulgur is used in salads, soups, casseroles, or ice cream to substitute nuts. It has a slightly different flavor than wheat berries. The shelf life is almost indefinite.

Whole wheat berries can also be put through a wheat grinder to make cracked wheat and whole wheat flour. Whole wheat can be cracked in a blender as well. The cracked wheat can be done in various sizes as desired for use. I like the small size of cracked wheat: it cooks faster and is easier to use as a meat substitute. Cracked wheat soaked in water for ½–2 hours and added to hamburger is a nutritious meat extender—1 part cracked wheat to 4 parts meat (½–1 cup cracked wheat to 1 pound hamburger).

Whole wheat berries can be soaked to make sprouts or cooked whole, making them chewy. The kernel will expand and with successive rinses, the soaked kernel will sprout.

Sprouting Wheat and Other Grains

1 Tbsp. sprouting seed

1 Tbsp. wheat berries or grains

Soak grain overnight if large grain. Drain well. Spread grain (single layer best) on cookie sheet using a shallow tray, plastic sprouter box, or even a plastic or glass jar. Keep moist—rinse 2–3 times a day with lukewarm water. Drain well. These are tender sprouts—cold or hot water could kill them. Store in a dark place until sprouts appear.

The sprouted wheat when exposed to the sun will turn green. This is known as wheat grass or sprouted wheat. The sprouted wheat can be used in candy, casseroles, desserts, salads, and even ground up for drinks. It is high in vitamin C. Sprouting seeds may take 4–7 days.

There are different ways you can cook wheat:

1 cup whole wheat

½ tsp. salt

2 cups boiling water

1. Simmer on lowest heat over water in double boiler overnight.

2. Bake overnight or for 5 hours at 150 degrees in a covered pan.

3. Put wheat, salt, and water in a quart-size thermos. Cover the top tightly and leave overnight.

4. Put ingredients in slow cooker. Set on low and leave all night.

Sift whole wheat flour 3 times to make lighter texture.

When making bread, use water instead of milk to make a light texture bread.

In using whole wheat in yeast breads, use more yeast or let it rise longer.

In using whole wheat with baking powder, increase baking powder by 1 teaspoon for each 3 cups of whole wheat flour. Recipes using baking soda do not need to be adjusted.

Mixing half whole wheat and half white flour sometimes gives a better result. You don't need to use 100 percent whole wheat flour all the time.

Soaking whole wheat flour in the liquid a few minutes before mixing can help prevent the bread from becoming crumbly when sliced.

One cup of soy flour can be substituted for one cup of whole wheat flour.

When baking whole wheat bread, add 1 tablespoon of vinegar or lemon juice for every tablespoon yeast. The acid tenderizes the gluten and makes the bread rise higher. This extends the life of the bread and keeps it soft without changing the flavor.

Whole wheat dough should nearly triple in size before it is ready to be punched down. White flour dough only doubles in size. Keep dough at 85 degrees during rising period for best results.

Whole wheat bread is likely to fall in the center during baking if the loaf pan is too wide on the bottom. Loaf pans used for white bread with a wide base are not as suitable for whole wheat dough. It is best to use the standard size pan, or smaller, having a width no wider than 3½ inches on the bottom.

To see if bread is done, wet your finger and touch the bottom of the bread pan. If it sizzles, the bread is done. You will not burn your finger. This works best with metal pans but also works with glass pans.

There are different types of whole wheat. One is white whole wheat, and this has all the nutrients and fiber of other whole wheat but will produce bread more white in color. This can be used in any recipe.

Everlasting Yeast: Stir 2 cups warm water in which potatoes have been cooked, ½ tablespoon yeast, 2 tablespoons flour, 1 tablespoon sugar, and 1 teaspoon salt. (Using a whole cake of yeast or 1 tablespoon dry yeast works best.) Put in warm place until ready to mix for baking. Leave small amount of everlasting yeast for a starter. Store in cool place until a few hours before ready to mix again. Mix and add to yeast mixture daily 1 teaspoon flour, 1 teaspoon sugar, ⅛ teaspoon salt. This is called feeding the mix. You will always have yeast on hand.

For ingredient lists, one package of yeast equals one tablespoon of yeast.

Breads and Crackers

Whole Wheat Bread

8 cups whole wheat flour
⅓ cup vegetable oil
⅓ cup honey or molasses
2 Tbsp. salt
4 Tbsp. lecithin granules (dough enhancer)
2 Tbsp. yeast dissolved in ½ cup warm water
6 cups warm water

Tip! Half the recipe if you're using a Kitchen Aid mixer.

Mix 4 cups of flour, oil, honey or molasses, salt, and lecithin granules. Mix in yeast mixture, then add water.

Knead 10 minutes. Add rest of flour. Knead 5 more minutes. Let rise until dough doubles in size. Mold into 2 loaf pans. Let rise again about ½ hour. Bake at 375 degrees for 45 minutes.

Basic Whole Wheat Bread

This recipe is for a bread maker.

2 cups warm water
2 cups whole wheat flour
2 cups white flour
2 Tbsp. margarine
2 Tbsp. vinegar
¼ cup sugar
1 tsp. salt
1½ Tbsp. yeast

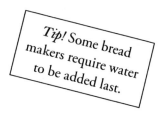

Tip! Some bread makers require water to be added last.

Put ingredients in bread maker in the above order. Bake at regular or wheat setting for bread.

Sweet Whole Wheat Bread

1 pkg. dry yeast
¼ cup hot water
½ cup brown sugar
1 tsp. salt
2½ cups lukewarm water
¼ cup shortening
3½ cup whole wheat flour
4 cups white flour

Dissolve yeast in water. In medium bowl, stir brown sugar and salt in lukewarm water until dissolved. Add shortening, whole wheat flour, and 1 cup white flour. Beat thoroughly. Stir in dissolved yeast. Add enough of the remaining flour to make a dough that leaves the sides of the bowl. Put on floured board, cover, and let rest 10–15 minutes. Knead until smooth and elastic, 5–7 minutes. Put in greased bowl and turn dough over to grease top. Cover and let rise until doubled in size, about 1½ hours. Punch dough down, and divide in half. Round up each half to make a ball. Cover and let rest 10 minutes. Shape into loaves and place in two greased loaf pans. Let rise until dough reaches top of pan on sides and the top of the loaf is well rounded above pans, about 80 minutes. Bake at 375 degrees for 45 minutes. Cover baking bread loosely with foil the last 20 minutes if necessary to prevent excessive browning.

Whole Wheat Loaf

2 cups cracked wheat
2 cups water
1½ cup whole wheat flour
1 tsp. salt
2 Tbsp. vegetable oil
2 Tbsp. butter

Soak cracked wheat in water and let sit at least 30 minutes. Mix in flour and salt. Press into a greased loaf pan and refrigerate at least 4 hours. Slice into 8–10 pieces. Fry slices in vegetable oil on medium to low heat in melted butter until crisp, both sides.

VARIATION: Add ¼ cup each of diced onion, diced celery, dried or fresh diced tomato, and 1 tablespoon beef base. Mix all together before pressing into loaf pan.

Makes 8 servings.

Sandwich Bread

2 cups milk
¼ cup margarine
½ cup brown sugar
1 egg
1½ tsp. salt
2 Tbsp. yeast
5 cups flour (white or mixed with wheat)

Heat milk and margarine until lukewarm. Pour in mixing bowl; add brown sugar, egg, salt, yeast, and 2 cups white flour. Mix 2 minutes with mixer, then add 3 more cups flour. Mix by hand. Let dough rise twice. Bake in two loaf pans. Bake at 375 degrees 40–45 minutes.

Freezer Whole Wheat Bread

1 cup milk
½ cup margarine
¼ cup sugar
½ cup brown sugar
2 tsp. salt
2¼ cups warm water
3 pkgs. dry yeast
3 cups whole wheat flour
7–8 cups white flour

Combine milk, margarine, sugar, brown sugar, and salt in a saucepan. Heat until margarine melts. Cool. In a large bowl, sprinkle yeast into water and stir. Add milk mixture, whole wheat flour, and 1 cup white flour. Beat until smooth. Stir in enough white flour to make dough stiff. Knead until smooth and elastic, about 10 minutes. Cover and let rest for 15 minutes. Divide dough into 3 parts. Line bread pans with aluminum foil or plastic wrap. Put dough into pans. Freeze.

To Bake: Take off foil or plastic wrap and put dough back in bread pans. Let rise until dough doubles in size. Bake at 375 degrees for 35 minutes.

Makes 3 loaves.

Easy Whole Wheat Bread

This is as easy as 1-2-3-(4)!

1 Tbsp. baking soda
2 cups brown sugar
3 cups buttermilk
4 cups whole wheat flour

Mix ingredients well and pour into 2 loaf pans. Bake at 325 degrees 50–60 minutes.

Optional: Bake in bread maker on quick bread setting.

Whole Grain Buttermilk Bread

2 pkgs. dry yeast
¼ cup warm water
2 cups buttermilk
¼ cup margarine
½ cup honey
2 tsp. salt
2 cups whole wheat flour
2 cups rye flour
2–3 cups white flour

Dissolve yeast in water. Heat margarine, honey, and salt in buttermilk until margarine melts. Add to yeast mixture in large bowl. Stir in wheat flour, rye flour, and 1 cup white flour until smooth. Beat in enough flour to make soft dough. Put into 2 greased loaf pans. Bake at 350 degrees for 45 minutes.

Quick Whole Wheat Nut Bread

¾ cup sugar
¼ cup shortening
2 eggs
½ tsp. cinnamon
1 cup white flour
2 tsp. baking powder
¼ tsp. salt
¼ tsp. allspice
¼ tsp. nutmeg
¼ cup milk
¼ tsp. vanilla
¼ cup chopped nuts

Cream sugar and shortening. Beat in eggs. Mix dry ingredients together. Stir in milk and vanilla to creamed mixture. Add nuts. Pour into greased loaf pan. Bake at 350 degrees for 45 minutes.

Whole Wheat Pumpkin Quick Bread

1½ cups sugar
½ cup melted butter
2 eggs
1 cup pumpkin, canned or fresh
½ cup water
½ tsp. ginger
1¼ cups white flour
¾ cup whole wheat flour
½ tsp. nutmeg
1 tsp. baking soda
¼ tsp. baking powder
½ tsp. salt
½ tsp. cinnamon
½ tsp. cloves ground
½ cup chopped walnuts

Cream sugar and butter together. Add eggs, pumpkin, and water; mix thoroughly. Sift dry ingredients together; add to pumpkin mixture. Stir until moist. Add walnuts. Pour into greased loaf pan. Bake at 350 degrees for 70 minutes. Remove from pan and cool on wire rack. Cool thoroughly before slicing.

Whole Wheat Potato Bread

1¾ cups white flour
2 pkgs. dry yeast
1 cup milk
½ cup water
2 Tbsp. butter
2 Tbsp. sugar
1 Tbsp. salt
1½ cups seasoned mashed potatoes
½ cup sour cream
½ cup minced onion
2 tsp. tarragon
1 tsp. garlic powder (optional)
5-6 cups whole wheat flour

Stir together white flour and yeast. Blend milk, water, butter, sugar, and salt over low heat until warm. Add liquid ingredients to flour and yeast and beat until smooth, about 3 minutes. Beat in potatoes, sour cream, onion, tarragon, and garlic powder until smooth. Stir in enough flour to make moderately stiff dough. Put on floured surface; let rise until double in size, about 45 minutes. Punch down. Divide dough in half and shape into two loaves. Put in greased loaf pans. Let dough rise again until almost doubled in size, about 30 minutes. Bake at 375 degrees 35–40 minutes.

Quick Wheat Banana Bread

1¼ cup white flour
1 cup whole wheat flour
1½ tsp. baking powder
½ tsp. baking soda
½ tsp. salt
½ tsp. nutmeg
½ cup softened margarine
½ cup sugar
2 eggs
1 cup mashed ripe bananas
¼ cup buttermilk
½ cup chopped walnuts
¼ cup finely snipped dried apricots

Blend flours, baking powder, baking soda, salt, and nutmeg. Cream margarine and sugar; beat in eggs. Add dry ingredients to creamed mixture. Blend in banana and buttermilk. Stir in walnuts and apricots. Pour batter into greased loaf pan. Bake at 350 degrees 50–60 minutes or until a toothpick inserted in the middle comes out clean. Cool in pan for 10 minutes. Remove from pan and continue to cool on wire rack. Wrap in plastic wrap or foil and store 8–10 hours before slicing.

Irish Brown Soda Bread

3 cups whole wheat flour
1½ cups sifted white flour
1 tsp. salt
1 tsp. baking soda
1 Tbsp. sugar
1 Tbsp. soft margarine
1½–1⅔ cups buttermilk*

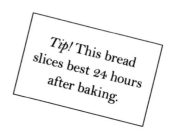

Tip! This bread slices best 24 hours after baking.

Preheat oven to 425 degrees. Sift together the flours, salt, baking soda, and sugar. Cream in the margarine. Add buttermilk gradually until the dough is soft but not sticky. Form dough into a ball and knead in the bowl with floured hands. Do not overknead. Place on a lightly greased baking sheet and flatten it with your palm into a circle 1½ inches thick. Cut a cross on the top to prevent cracking during baking. Bake for 25 minutes, then reduce heat to 350 degrees and bake 15 more minutes. Cool on a wire rack; seal tightly in a plastic bag.

*Substitute: 6 tablespoons vinegar with 1½ cups milk equals 1½ cups buttermilk.

No Knead Bread

2 cups warm water
2½ Tbsp. margarine
2 tsp. salt
1½ Tbsp. yeast
2½ Tbsp. sugar
1 egg
2½ cups whole wheat flour
2½ cups white flour

Mix ingredients together and knead if desired. Place in an airtight container. The container has to be at least double the size of the dough. The warm air trapped helps the bread to rise faster. Let rise 30 minutes. Put into two loaf pans. Let rise again 30 minutes. Bake at 350 degrees for 30 minutes.

Note: If you want to double the recipe, some measurements and ingredients change.

3¾ cups warm water
⅓ cup oil
4 tsp. salt
3 Tbsp. yeast
⅓ cup sugar
2 eggs
5 cups white flour
5 cups whole wheat flour

Ninety-Minute Whole Wheat Bread

1 cup warm water
2 Tbsp. yeast
2 Tbsp. brown sugar
⅓ cup honey
1 Tbsp. salt
3 cups warm water
1 cup instant milk powder*
8 cups whole wheat flour

Mix 1 cup warm water, yeast, and brown sugar; let stand 5 minutes. Mix honey, salt, 3 cups warm water, and instant milk powder. Add flour and stir well. Grease three 46-oz. empty juice cans. Divide dough into 3 parts and put in cans. Place cans standing up in oven. Bake at 350 degrees for 1 minute. Turn oven off let bread raise in oven for 15 minutes. Bake at 350 degrees for 50 minutes. Cool bread in cans for 10 minutes. Put on rack to finish cooling.

*If milk is non-instant, use only ½ cup plus 3 tablespoons flour to avoid lumping.

French Bread

5½–6 cups flour (may use 2 cups of whole wheat flour)
3 tsp. salt
1 Tbsp. sugar
2 Tbsp. yeast
2 Tbsp. shortening
2 cups warm water
1 egg white
1–2 Tbsp. water

Mix all ingredients; let rise until double in size. Punch down and roll into shapes, such as hogi rolls or hamburger buns. Place on greased sheet and let them double in size. Mix egg white and water; brush on dough. Bake at 375 degrees 35–40 minutes.

Anadama Bread

This is always a favorite for first-timers.

½ cup yellow cornmeal
½ cup boiling water
1 Tbsp. yeast
½ cup warm water
¼ cup dark molasses
2 Tbsp. butter
1 tsp. salt
3 cups white flour

Mix cornmeal in boiling water. Let stand until cool. Dissolve the yeast in the warm water in a large bowl. Let stand until yeast foams, about 5 minutes. Add molasses, butter, salt, and cooled cornmeal mixture. Stir in half the flour. Beat well. Add more flour, beating until dough is stiff. Cover and let stand 15 minutes. Put dough on a floured surface. Knead 5 minutes or until smooth and elastic. Put dough in greased bowl and cover. Let rise until doubled in size, about 1 hour. Punch down and shape into a ball. Grease two loaf pans. Place dough in pans, smooth side up. Let rise until doubled in size, about 1 hour. Bake at 375 degrees 30–35 minutes.

Whole Wheat Buns

2 cups whole wheat flour
2½ cups white flour
2 pkgs. dry yeast
2 Tbsp. margarine, softened
2 eggs
1 (12-oz.) pkg. cottage cheese
1½ Tbsp. dill seed
2 tsp. salt
¼ cup sugar
2 tsp. dehydrated onion, soaked in a very small amount of water
½ cup lukewarm water

Mix wheat flour, 1½ cups white flour, and yeast. Add margarine, eggs, and cottage cheese. Stir in dill seed, salt, sugar, and onion. Add water and beat for 2 minutes at medium speed, scraping the bowl often. Mix in 1 cup of white flour; add enough flour to make a smooth dough. Put on lightly floured surface and knead until smooth and elastic (it may be sticky). Put in greased bowl; turn it over to grease top. Cover and let rise until double in size, about 1 hour. Punch down; let rest 10 minutes. Divide into 24 balls. Place on greased baking sheet. Press down to form a bun. Let buns rise until double in size. Bake at 400 degrees 10–15 minutes or until brown. Remove from pans and cool on wire rack.

VARIATION: For flat hamburger style buns, grease the bottom of a cookie sheet and put on top of buns while they are rising. Remove before baking.

Makes 2 dozen buns.

Refrigerator Rolls

2 cups warm water
2 Tbsp. yeast
½ cup sugar
2 tsp. salt
¼ cup shortening
1 egg
3 cups whole wheat flour
3½–4 cups white flour

Put yeast in warm water and set aside. Cream sugar, salt, and shortening. Blend in egg. Add whole wheat flour and 3½ cups white flour. Mix in the yeast mixture. Dough should be smooth and come away from bowl. If it is sticky, add more white flour. Cover with a damp towel or wax paper. Refrigerate until ready to use.

When you want to make rolls, take out the amount of dough you need, divide into balls, shape, and put on greased cookie sheet. Allow to rise until double in size. Bake at 400 degrees 12–15 minutes. This dough can be refrigerated up to five days.

Whole Wheat Parker House Rolls

¼ cup shortening
2 Tbsp. sugar
¾ tsp. salt
½ cup boiling water
1 pkg. yeast
1 tsp. sugar
½ cup warm water
1 egg, slightly beaten
1 cup whole wheat flour
1½ cups white flour
½ cup graham cracker crumbs
melted butter or margarine

Combine shortening, sugar, salt, and boiling water; cool to luke-warm. Dissolve yeast and 1 teaspoon sugar in ½ cup warm water. Add yeast mixture and egg to shortening mixture. Stir in flours and cracker crumbs, blending well. Place in a greased bowl; turn over to grease top. Cover and let rise in warm place until it doubles in size. Roll dough to ¼-inch thickness; cut into 2½-inch rounds with a biscuit cutter. With dull edge of knife, press a crease just off center of each round, making the dough more oval; brush with melted butter. Fold edges over so they overlap and press together. Place on greased baking sheets. Let rise in a warm place until doubled in size. Bake at 350 degrees 15–20 minutes.

Makes 2 dozen.

VARIATIONS

Crescent Rolls: Roll dough into a circle, then cut 12 pie-shaped pieces. Roll the pieces from the large end to the small end and bake as above.

Cloverleaf Rolls: Put smooth balls of dough in greased muffin tin. Cut a cross on top of dough. Or, make three small balls and place them in a greased muffin tin.

Quick Baking Powder Biscuits

2 cups whole wheat flour
1 Tbsp. sugar
1 tsp. salt
4 tsp. baking powder
¼ cup shortening
⅔ cup milk

Mix dry ingredients, then cut in shortening. Add enough of the milk to make soft dough. On floured surface, press or roll to ½-inch thick and cut in desired shapes. Bake at 400 degrees for 15 minutes.

Makes 1 dozen.

Pita Bread

2 Tbsp. dry yeast
¼ tsp. salt
½ cup warm water
1½ Tbsp. salt
¼ cup oil
5 cups whole wheat flour

Dissolve yeast and ¼ teaspoon salt in water. Add the rest of the salt and oil. Mix in one cup of flour at a time. Put on floured surface and knead for 10 minutes. Put in greased bowl and turn over to grease top. Let rise for 1–1½ hours. Punch down and let rest for 10 minutes. Divide into 12 balls. Cover and let rest for 3 minutes. Roll each piece into 7-inch diameter circles. Grease and sprinkle baking sheets with cornmeal. Put dough on sheets; cover and let rest for 30 minutes. Bake at 450 degrees for 5 minutes on top rack of oven. Move to bottom rack and bake for another 5 minutes.

Makes 1 dozen.

Basic Wheat Pretzels

2 cups whole wheat flour
2 cups white flour
1 pkg. dry yeast
1 tsp. salt
3 Tbsp. vegetable oil
1⅓ cups hot water
coarse salt

Preheat oven to 425 degrees. Grease large baking sheet. Stir together whole wheat and white flour. Combine 1½ cups of mixed flours with yeast and salt. Add oil and water and beat until smooth, about 2 minutes. Add more flour as needed to make moderately stiff dough. Knead 3–5 minutes or until smooth. Divide into 12 pieces and roll each into a ¾-inch thick, 10-inch long rope. Shape into an upside-down U, bring ends to top of U, cross, and press to dough. Place on greased baking sheet and sprinkle salt on top. Bake for 20 minutes or until light brown.

Makes 1 dozen.

Seasoned Whole Wheat Pretzels

1 Tbsp. yeast
1½ cups warm water
1 Tbsp. caraway seeds
½ tsp. anise seed
½ tsp. salt
2 tsp. malted milk powder*
1 Tbsp. molasses
3 cups whole wheat flour
coarse salt
1 egg white

Preheat oven to 425 degrees. Put yeast in warm water while mixing other ingredients. Mix all ingredients except coarse salt and egg white, then add yeast mixture and knead 15 minutes. Divide into 12 pieces and roll each into a ¾-inch thick, 10-inch long rope. Dip in water, shape into an upside-down U, bring ends to top of U, cross, and press to dough. Place on greased cookie sheet and sprinkle with coarse salt. Bake 10 minutes. Brush with egg white and bake 5–10 minutes or until brown.

*Milk powder can be used if you can't find malted milk powder.

Makes 1 dozen.

Whole Wheat Crackers

4 cups whole wheat flour
2 tsp. salt
⅔ cup milk
⅓ cup vegetable oil
1 Tbsp. honey
1½ cups warm water
1 Tbsp. yeast

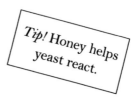

Tip! Honey helps yeast react.

Mix ingredients and cover bowl. Let rise until it doubles in size, usually ½–1 hour. Roll part of dough on floured surface until very thin. Put on cookie sheet. Score into any desired cracker shapes. Bake at 350 degrees for 20 minutes or until golden brown. Cool on wire rack; break carefully or cut with scissors. Store in airtight container.

Makes about 5 dozen, depending on size.

Thick Wheat Crackers

1¼ cups white flour
1¼ cups whole wheat flour
¼ tsp. baking soda
1½ tsp. salt
¼ cup shortening
¼ cup yogurt
¼ tsp. coarse salt

Stir together flours, baking soda, regular salt, and shortening until mixture is crumbly. Gently stir yogurt in with a fork. Press and shape into a ball. Wrap and chill until dough is stiff. Roll out to ½-inch thick; cut into shapes and sprinkle with coarse salt. Lift with a spatula onto cookie sheet. Bake at 400 degrees 5–7 minutes. Place on wire rack to cool. Store in airtight container.

Makes about 5 dozen, depending on size.

Wheat Crackers Variation

⅓ cup vegetable oil
¾ Tbsp. salt
¾ cup water
1¾ cups whole wheat flour
1½ cups white flour
coarse salt

Whip oil. Add salt and water. Mix in flours. Roll out to ⅛-inch thick on cookie sheet. Score into shapes and prick each one. Sprinkle with coarse salt. Bake at 350 degrees or until light brown and crispy. Place on wire rack and cut with scissors or break carefully when cool. Store in airtight container.

Makes 5 dozen, depending on size.

Oatmeal Crackers

½ cup shortening
¼ cup butter or margarine, softened
½ cup sugar
3 cups whole wheat flour
2 cups rolled oats
1½ tsp. salt
1½ cups milk

Cream shortening, butter, and sugar until fluffy. In large bowl, stir together flour, oats, and salt; set aside. Gradually combine creamed ingredients, flour mixture, and milk. Dough will be soft and sticky. Knead lightly on floured surface. Divide into four parts, wrap, and refrigerate for several hours. On floured surface, roll out each piece ⅛-inch thick. Cut with cookie cutter. Prick all over with fork; put on cookie sheets. Bake at 350 degrees 20–25 minutes or until golden brown. Cool on racks.

Makes 5 dozen, depending on size.

Graham Crackers

½ cup margarine
⅔ cup brown sugar
2¾ cups whole wheat flour
¼ tsp. cinnamon
½ tsp. baking powder
½ cup water

Cream together margarine and brown sugar. Add flour, cinnamon, and baking powder. Gradually add water. Let stand 30 minutes. Roll ⅛-inch thick. Cut in squares and bake on greased cookie sheet at 350 degrees for 20 minutes.

Makes 3 dozen, depending on size.

Graham Crackers Variation

3 cups whole wheat flour
¾ tsp. baking soda
1 tsp. baking powder
½ tsp. salt
3 Tbsp. butter
1 tsp. vanilla
⅔ cup brown sugar
3 Tbsp. vegetable oil
2 Tbsp. honey
2 Tbsp. molasses
½ cup sour cream

Mix all ingredients except sour cream. Then blend in sour cream. Sprinkle cookie sheet with flour. Roll out dough until thin on cookie sheet, or between two sheets of wax paper and then put on cookie sheet. Use a pizza cutter or knife to score into squares. Bake at 375 degrees 6–8 minutes.

Makes 4 dozen, depending on size.

Seasoned Crackers

2 cups cool water
1 tsp. garlic powder
1 tsp. onion powder
1 tsp. salt
2 cups whole wheat flour
sesame seeds (optional)

Mix water, garlic and onion powders, and salt in blender. Slowly add flour. Blend until flour is just mixed. Pour batter in a squirt catsup bottle and squirt onto greased cookie sheet. Sprinkle on sesame seeds. Bake at 350 degrees for 15 minutes.

Makes 3 dozen, depending on size.

Croutons

30–33 slices whole wheat bread cut in ½-inch cubes
⅓ cup vegetable oil
¾ tsp. ground sage
3 Tbsp. minced onion
3 Tbsp. dried parsley flakes
2 tsp. garlic salt
½ tsp. seasoned pepper
1 tsp. each thyme, marjoram, basil

Preheat oven to 300 degrees. Toast bread cubes on cookie sheet for ½ hour. Raise temperature to 325 degrees and bake until brown, stirring occasionally. Remove from oven and add the rest of the ingredients. Mix well and store in airtight container.

Makes 1 gallon.

Whole Wheat Noodles

5½ cups whole wheat flour
3 medium eggs
1½ cups hot water, as needed

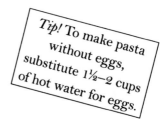

Tip! To make pasta without eggs, substitute 1½–2 cups of hot water for eggs.

Mix flour and eggs in large bowl with a wooden spoon or floured hands until the dough can be gathered into a ball. Moisten dough with water if necessary. Put dough on floured surface. Knead dough until smooth and elastic, 3–5 minutes. Cut into four pieces. Roll each piece flat into a small rectangle.

These can be cut and used immediately or frozen. Stored as rectangles, they take much less freezer space than bags of noodles.

Pizza Dough

Make a deep-dish pizza in a square pan by having dough on the sides.

½ cup water
1 Tbsp. olive oil
1 tsp. salt
1 cup white flour
½ cup whole wheat flour
1 pkg. yeast

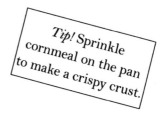

Tip! Sprinkle cornmeal on the pan to make a crispy crust.

Heat water, oil, and salt until salt is dissolved. Cool to lukewarm. Add flours and yeast. Knead well; let it rise until it doubles in size. Punch down and let rest 10 minutes. Roll out into a 9-inch diameter and place on pizza pan or greased cookie sheet, or pat into a 9 x 9 greased pan. Slightly grease the top. Add your favorite pizza toppings and bake at 425 degrees, until cheese melts or crust is slightly brown.

Breakfast

Waffles and Pancakes

1 cup wheat flour
¼ tsp. salt
3 tsp. baking powder
2 tsp. sugar
2 eggs
1¼ cups milk
3 Tbsp. vegetable oil or melted shortening

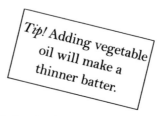

Tip! Adding vegetable oil will make a thinner batter.

Mix dry ingredients. Gradually add eggs and milk, mixing at a slow speed. Mix in vegetable oil. Bake in preheated waffle iron. For pancakes, use ½ cup additional whole wheat flour.

Makes 4 waffles or 6 pancakes.

Whole Wheat Pancakes

⅓ cup vegetable oil
4½ tsp. baking powder
4 cups milk
1 tsp. salt
3 cups whole wheat flour
4 egg whites

Mix all the ingredients except egg whites. In a separate bowl, beat egg whites until stiff, then fold into batter. Bake on griddle.

Makes 14–16.

Best Ever Pancakes

This is a favorite for breakfast and very easy.

¾ cup whole wheat berries
1 cup milk
3 eggs
½ cup vegetable oil
1 Tbsp. honey
2 tsp. baking powder
1 tsp. baking soda
1 tsp. salt

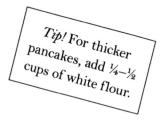

Tip! For thicker pancakes, add ¼–½ cups of white flour.

In blender, blend wheat berries and milk on high for 4 minutes. Refrigerate overnight. Add eggs, vegetable oil, honey, baking powder, baking soda, and salt. Blend in blender about 5 minutes or until mostly smooth. Grill batter on hot frying pan.

Makes 10–12.

Whole Wheat Blender Pancakes

You will be surprised at how light and fluffy these pancakes are.

1 cup whole wheat
1½ cups milk
½ cup vegetable oil
2 tsp. sugar
1 tsp. salt
1 egg
3 tsp. baking powder

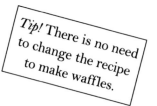

Tip! There is no need to change the recipe to make waffles.

In blender, blend whole wheat and 1 cup milk on high for at least 3 minutes. Add ½ cup milk and blend. Add rest of ingredients and blend until smooth. Cook on hot griddle.

Makes 4.

Potato Pancakes

These are traditionally served with applesauce.

3-4 cups potatoes, peeled, sliced, boiled
2 Tbsp. whole wheat flour
1-2 eggs
1 small onion, minced
salt to taste
vegetable oil

Grate or mash potatoes. Mix well with flour, eggs, onion, and salt. Drop by spoonful or ¼ measuring cup on hot greased pan and flatten them like a pancake. Fry on both sides until brown and crisp.

Makes 1 dozen.

Whole Wheat Waffles

1 cup whole wheat
1 cup milk
3 eggs
3 Tbsp. margarine
3 Tbsp. cornmeal
1 Tbsp. sugar
½ tsp. salt
1 tsp. baking powder

Blend wheat and milk in blender. Add eggs, margarine, cornmeal, sugar, and salt. Blend well. Mix in baking powder. Cook on waffle iron.

Makes 10–12.

Night-Before French Toast

1 loaf whole wheat bread, unsliced
8 eggs, beaten
1 tsp. vanilla
3 cups milk
3 tsp. sugar
¾ tsp. salt
4–6 Tbsp. margarine

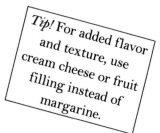

Tip! For added flavor and texture, use cream cheese or fruit filling instead of margarine.

Grease loaf pan. Cut bread in 1-inch slices and arrange in pan. Beat eggs with vanilla, milk, sugar, and salt. Pour over bread. Dot top with margarine. Cover with plastic wrap and refrigerate 4–6 hours or overnight. Bake at 350 degrees for 40 minutes or until bread is puffy and lightly browned. Remove from oven and let cool a few minutes. Cut and serve with syrup or fruit.

Makes 10–12 servings.

Quick-and-Easy Breakfast Toast

This imitation of a pancake is unbelievably good!

1 thick slice whole wheat bread
butter
syrup

Toast bread. Top with butter and syrup on toast.

Makes 1 serving.

Hot Cereal

¼ cup quick-cooking oatmeal
¼ cup cracked wheat
1 cup water
⅛ tsp. salt

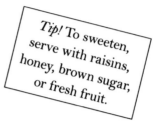

Tip! To sweeten, serve with raisins, honey, brown sugar, or fresh fruit.

Put ingredients in a cereal bowl and microwave for 1½ minutes. You may want to put the bowl on a plate in case it spills. (Timing will depend on your microwave.)

Makes 1 serving.

Hot Cereal for the Family

Try doubling the recipe and cooking it in a slow cooker on low overnight, and it will be ready in the morning!

1 cup cracked wheat
1 cup quick-cooking oatmeal
7 cups water
1½ tsp. salt
2 Tbsp. margarine

Combine all ingredients in medium saucepan and bring to a boil. Simmer 10–20 minutes or until thick.

Makes 10 servings.

Whole Wheat Cereal

This is the basic recipe for cooked wheat.

1 cup whole wheat
½ tsp. salt
2 cups boiling water

Serve with honey, brown sugar, and milk.

Makes 2 servings.

Cream of Wheat

¼ cup wheat flour
¼ cup sugar (or less)
2 cups milk
2 eggs

Stove Top: Cook flour, sugar, and milk over low heat, stirring occasionally every 3–4 minutes. Take a small amount of the hot cereal out, put in small bowl, and beat in 2 eggs. Gradually add egg mixture back into cereal. This prevents eggs from cooking before being blended with cereal. Cook 2 more minutes.

Microwave: Combine flour, sugar, and milk and microwave for 6 minutes. Stir and microwave 4 more minutes. Take a small amount of the hot cereal out, put in small bowl, and beat in 2 eggs. Gradually add egg mixture back into cereal. This prevents eggs from cooking before being blended with cereal. Microwave 4–6 more minutes. Allow to cool before eating.

Makes 4 servings.

Wheat Cereal

6 cups whole wheat flour
½ tsp. salt
2 cups buttermilk*
1 tsp. baking soda
1½ cups brown sugar

Mix ingredients thoroughly. Press or roll evenly onto two cookie sheets. Bake at 350 degrees until golden brown on edges. Turn oven down to 200 degrees. Take out cereal and turn it over with spatula, breaking cereal into small pieces. Return to oven to dry out.

When cooled, grind chunks in food processor. Sift out small granular pieces. Larger pieces may be used for cereal or casseroles. Smaller pieces may be used for pie crusts and other desserts.

VARIATIONS
Sweet: Add cinnamon or nutmeg before baking to give a custard or eggnog flavor.

Poultry Stuffing: Eliminate sugar and add sage, poultry seasoning, celery salt, and bouillon cubes.

Salad Toppers: Add garlic salt, onion powder, salt, or other favorite spices.

Dog or Cat Food: Reduce sugar and add bouillon. Break up chunks for the appropriate size.

Makes 5 cups cereal or 2 cups crumbs.

*Substitute: 2 cups milk plus 2 tablespoons vinegar or lemon juice.

Granola With Fruit

2½ cups quick-cooking oatmeal
½ cup sesame seeds
½ cup sunflower seeds, shelled
1 cup shredded coconut
½ cup wheat germ
½ cup honey
½ cup vegetable oil
½ cup raisins
½ cup dried apricots, chopped

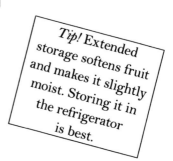

Tip! Extended storage softens fruit and makes it slightly moist. Storing it in the refrigerator is best.

Preheat oven to 300 degrees. Mix everything except the apricots and raisins and spread in 9 x 13 pan. Bake until light golden brown, or about 45 minutes. Stir every 15 minutes. Remove from oven and stir in dried apricots and raisins. Remove to another pan to cool. Stir occasionally during cooling to prevent lumping. Store in tightly covered jars or plastic bags.

Makes 6½ cups.

Sweet Granola

4 cups quick-cooking oatmeal
2½ cups wheat germ
1 tsp. cinnamon
½ cup honey
⅔ cup vegetable oil
2 Tbsp. vanilla
2 Tbsp. brown sugar
1 cup coconut, raisins, sunflower seeds, dried fruit (use 1 cup each or use 1 cup total)

Preheat oven to 300 degrees. Mix ingredients in large bowl and spread on cookie sheet. Bake about 20 minutes or until slightly brown. Stir occasionally during baking.

Makes 6–8 servings.

Muesli

Try this for a healthy breakfast cereal.

4 cups quick-cooking oatmeal
1 cup chopped nuts
1 cup crunchy wheat cereal
1 cup dried apples
1 cup apricots
1 cup raisins
1 cup wheat bran

Mix together and put in covered container.

Makes 6 servings.

Buttermilk Muffins

2 cups buttermilk*
2 cups cracked wheat
½ cup margarine
½ cup brown sugar
1 egg
½ tsp. salt
1 cup flour (whole wheat or white)
2 tsp. baking soda
1 tsp. baking powder
½ cup raisins, chopped dates, or chopped walnuts

Mix buttermilk and cracked wheat; set aside. Cream margarine and sugar. Mix in wheat mixture. Add egg and salt and mix. Refrigerate overnight or at least 6 hours.

Mix in flour, baking soda, and baking powder. Add raisins, dates, or walnuts. Put in two greased loaf pans. Bake at 400 degrees for 20 minutes or until a knife comes out clean.

*Substitute: 2 cups milk plus 2 tablespoons vinegar.

Quick Whole Wheat Bread and Muffins

1 cup milk
1 egg
½ cup oil
½ cup honey
¼ tsp. salt
3 tsp. baking powder
2 cups whole wheat flour

Mix wet ingredients in small bowl. Mix dry ingredients in medium bowl. Mix in wet ingredients. For bread, pour into a greased loaf pan and bake at 350 degrees for 45 minutes. For muffins, pour into a greased muffin tin and bake at 350 degrees for 25 minutes.

Makes 1 dozen.

VARIATION: Add 2 teaspoons cinnamon and 1 cup blueberries, raisins, or other dried fruit.

Whole Wheat Muffins

4 cups whole wheat flour
1 cup cooking oil
2 eggs
2 cups milk
2 cups brown sugar
1 tsp. salt
2 tsp. baking soda
2 tsp. vanilla

Put whole wheat flour in large bowl. Mix other ingredients in medium bowl and pour mixture over flour. Mix well. Pour into greased muffin tins and bake at 375 degrees for 20 minutes.

Makes 2 dozen.

Soups and Salads

Minestrone Soup

2 Tbsp. vegetable oil
¾ cup chopped onions
1 lb. ground beef
1 cup chopped celery
6 cups water
1 cup cooked wheat berries
½ cup shredded cabbage
½ cup minced parsley
⅔ cup sliced carrots
1 cup kidney beans
1½ tsp. salt
¼ tsp. pepper
¼ tsp. oregano
1 can green beans or peas
1 cup sliced zucchini
parmesan cheese
croutons

In a large pot, sauté beef and onions in oil until onions are transparent and beef is browned. Drain grease. Add celery and water; cover and simmer slowly until celery is tender. Add wheat berries, cabbage, parsley, and carrots; cover and simmer 15 minutes. Add beans, salt and pepper, oregano, beans or peas, and zucchini. Simmer 15 minutes. Serve hot with parmesan cheese and croutons on top.

Makes 24 servings.

Cream of Potato Soup

1 cup boiling water
2 medium potatoes, peeled and diced
½ small onion diced
1 stalk celery diced
1 tsp. salt
1 Tbsp. butter
1 Tbsp. whole wheat flour
1½ cups milk

Add potatoes, onion, celery, and salt to boiling water. Cook until tender. In separate pan, melt butter. Stir in flour until mixture is smooth and thick. Add milk and vegetables. Stir or mash to make desired consistency for soup.

Makes 8 servings.

VARIATIONS: Add ¼ cup shredded cheddar cheese, ¼ cup cooked diced ham, or ¼ cup crushed red pepper flakes.

Wheat and Bean Chili

1 cup dry beans
1 cup wheat berries, uncooked
4 cups water
1 onion, chopped
3 Tbsp. vegetable oil
1 tsp. chili powder (to taste)
2 cups tomatoes
2 Tbsp. brown sugar
salt and pepper to taste

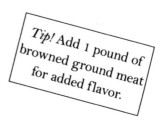

Tip! Add 1 pound of browned ground meat for added flavor.

Cook beans and wheat in water until tender in water. You can cook wheat and beans overnight in slow cooker. Add more water if needed. Sauté onion with oil. Add chili powder, tomatoes, brown sugar, and salt and pepper. Simmer one hour.

Makes 10 servings.

Wheat Chili

This chili tastes best the next day.

2 cups whole wheat
6 cups water
3 cubes beef bouillon
1 tsp. salt
1½ Tbsp. chili powder
1 large onion, chopped
4 cups canned tomatoes
1 (24-oz.) can tomato juice
¾ cup catsup

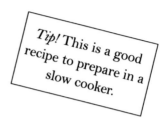

Tip! This is a good recipe to prepare in a slow cooker.

Wash wheat. Combine with water, bouillon cubes, and salt. Cook on low 2–3 hours. Add chili powder, onion, tomatoes, tomato juice, and catsup. Stir often to prevent sticking to the bottom of the pan. Remove from heat and let stand at room temperature for 6 hours, then overnight in refrigerator.

Makes 6 servings.

VARIATION: Brown 1 pound ground beef. Add beef and 1 cup beans to the remainder of the ingredients. Simmer 4–5 hours.

Wheat Seafood Salad

1 cup cracked wheat
½ cup French dressing
¼ cup chopped green onions
2 cups cold water
2–3 Tbsp. mayonnaise
¾ cup diced celery
½ tsp. salt
2 Tbsp. diced green pepper
1 cup tuna or shrimp
1 tomato, cut in wedges

Gently toss all ingredients. Chill before serving.

Makes 6 servings.

Whole Wheat and Tuna Salad

2 cups whole wheat, cooked
1 (7-oz.) can tuna
½ cup salad dressing
¼ cup chopped celery
½ cup sour cream
2 Tbsp. lemon juice
¼ cup chopped green onions (optional)
1 bottle pimentos (optional)

Tip! Use the pimentos and green onions as decoration.

Mix everything together and serve on bed of lettuce.

Makes 6 servings.

Cracked Wheat and Bean Salad

Salad
¼ cup uncooked rice
¼ cup cracked wheat
1¼ cups water
2 (15-oz.) cans kidney beans, drained
1 (11-oz.) can corn, drained
½ cup chopped onions

Dressing
¼ cup lemon juice
1 Tbsp. red wine vinegar
2 tsp. lemon peel (zest)
¼ cup olive oil

Salad: Boil rice and cracked wheat in water. Simmer 15 minutes or until soft. Allow to cool. In a bowl, combine beans, corn, and onions. Add rice and cracked wheat.

Dressing: Mix ingredients. Drizzle dressing over salad. Chill before serving.

Makes 5 servings.

Tabbouleh

This is a Middle East recipe typically found in Lebanon.

½ cup cracked wheat
2 Tbsp. fresh lemon juice
1½ Tbsp. olive oil
½ cup finely chopped green onions
½ clove garlic
1 tomato, diced
1¼ cups finely chopped celery
¾ cup finely chopped fresh parsley
1 cup finely chopped cucumber, seeded
½ tsp. salt

Stir cracked wheat, lemon juice, and olive oil in large bowl. Layer green onions, garlic, tomato, celery, parsley, and cucumber over cracked wheat mixture. Sprinkle salt. Cover and chill 24 hours. Toss well before serving.

Makes 6 servings.

Tip! Follow the order for the layers. The salt pulls water out of the vegetables, which in turn softens the cracked wheat as it chills overnight.

Vegetables and Side Dishes

Scalloped Potatoes

6 cups potatoes, peeled, boiled, and sliced thin
¼ cup finely chopped onion
1½ tsp. salt
dash of pepper
⅓ cup whole wheat flour
2 cups milk
2 Tbsp. butter
¼ cup fine whole wheat bread crumbs

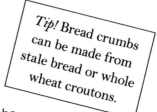

Tip! Bread crumbs can be made from stale bread or whole wheat croutons.

Place half of the potatoes in greased 2-qt. casserole dish. Add half the onion. Add salt and pepper to flour and sift over potatoes and onions. Repeat layers. Pour milk over mixture. Dot with butter and bread crumbs.

Makes 8 servings.

Golden Cheese Fondue

3 egg whites
1 Tbsp. butter
1 cup milk
1 cup whole wheat bread crumbs
1 cup cheddar cheese cubed
½ tsp. salt
⅛ tsp. black pepper

Beat egg whites until stiff. In a separate bowl, combine rest of the ingredients. Fold egg whites into mixture. Bake in 1½-qt. casserole dish at 350 degrees 35–40 minutes.

Makes 6 servings.

Cracked Wheat Pilaf

2 cups cracked wheat
5 cups beef broth
1 medium onion, chopped
¼ cup fresh parsley, minced, or 2 Tbsp. dried
¼ cup butter melted

Mix ingredients in a slow cooker. Cover and cook on high 3–4 hours or low 10–12 hours, stirring occasionally.

Makes 6 servings.

Wheat Pilaf

2 cups broth (vegetable or beef)
1 cup whole wheat berries
1 cup fresh green beans, cut in 1-inch pieces
1 onion, chopped
1 cup sliced mushrooms
1 tsp. thyme
1 tsp. marjoram or sage
salt and pepper to taste

Boil broth and wheat in a pot until tender. Add the rest of the ingredients and bring back to a boil. Cover and simmer 20–25 minutes, or until green beans are cooked. Remove from heat and let stand covered another 10 minutes.

Makes 6 servings.

Whole Wheat Cheesy Custard

2 eggs
2 cups grated cheese
¼ cup olive oil
2 cups cooked wheat
1 medium onion, grated
1 cup milk
¼ cup fresh parsley, or 1 tsp. dried
1 tsp. salt

Beat eggs until thick; add grated cheese. Add the rest of the ingredients. Mix well. Pour into greased casserole dish. Bake at 350 degrees for 1 hour. Let set 5–10 minutes.

Makes 6 servings.

Main Dishes

Triple Meat Loaf

½ lb. ground beef
½ lb. ground turkey
½ cup cracked wheat
¼ cup chopped onion
1 (8-oz.) can tomato sauce*
1 egg
2 tsp. parsley

Mix all ingredients and bake in loaf pan at 350 degrees 45–60 minutes.

*Substitute: Combine ½ can tomato sauce, 2 tablespoons mustard, 3 tablespoons brown sugar, 2 tablespoons vinegar, and 1 cup water.

Makes 8 servings.

Meat Loaf

1½ cups whole wheat bread crumbs
1 cup tomato juice or milk
1 large onion, chopped, or ¼ cup onion soup mix
½ tsp. pepper
2 tsp. salt
2 lb. ground beef
2 eggs
½ cup catsup or tomato soup
3 thin strips of bacon

Soak bread in milk or tomato juice for 10 minutes. Squeeze liquid out of bread and discard liquid. Mix all ingredients and shape in loaf pan. Top with ½ cup catsup or tomato soup and bacon. Bake at 325 degrees for 1½ hours.

Wheat Bean Burgers

1 cup cooked wheat
1 cup red kidney beans, cooked
1 tsp. beef base
meat seasonings

Blend wheat with food chopper, blender, or food processor. Drain beans and mash; save bean juice. Blend beans with wheat and seasonings and form patties; moisten with bean juice if necessary. Fry in skillet until browned and serve with catsup, soy sauce, or steak sauce.

Cracked Wheat Sausage

Unless you tell them, they'll never know these aren't real!
1 cup cooked cracked wheat
1½ tsp. sage
2–3 dashes onion salt
2–3 dashes garlic salt
1 beef bouillon cube
1 tsp. Worcestershire sauce
1 tsp. brown sugar
1 egg
3–4 drops Liquid Smoke

Mix ingredients and form into patties. If sausage is too moist, add oatmeal or bread crumbs. Fry with oil.

Makes 6 servings.

Meatballs

8 slices whole wheat bread, soaked in water
2 lbs. ground beef
4 eggs
1 cup grated parmesan cheese
¼ cup parsley
2 cloves garlic, minced
1 tsp. oregano
2 Tbsp. salt
⅛ tsp. black pepper

Squeeze water out of the bread; discard water. Mix ingredients and form into small balls. Bake at 350 degrees for 1 hour.

Makes 2 dozen.

Wheat Balls with Tomato

1 cup medium cracked wheat
¾ cup lukewarm water
1 cup whole wheat flour
3 Tbsp. beef base
1 can chick peas, drained and mashed
2 tsp. salt
½ cup vegetable oil
½ cup chopped onions
1 Tbsp. tomato paste (optional)

Soak wheat in water 5 minutes. Drain. Mix wheat, ¾ cup water, flour, beef base, chick peas, and 1 teaspoon salt; let set for 5 minutes. Boil saucepan of 8 cups of water and 1 teaspoon salt. Form small balls with moistened hands and drop into boiling water. Bring back to boil; simmer 25–30 minutes. Drain water, setting boiled water aside. Fry onion in oil until brown. Put onions over boiled wheat balls. Mix tomato paste with boiled water enough to make thin sauce and put over wheat balls. If you don't use tomato paste, squeeze lemon juice on top.

Makes 6 servings.

Sweet and Sour Meatballs

Meatballs
1 lb. ground beef
½ lb. sausage
1 tsp. soy sauce
1 clove minced garlic
¾ cup cooked cracked wheat

Sauce
1 (8-oz.) can crushed pineapple
1 (5-oz.) can water chestnuts, drained and diced
½ cup brown sugar
2 tsp. soy sauce
1 bouillon cube
2 tablespoons cornstarch combined with 1 cup water
½ tsp. salt
3 Tbsp. vinegar

Meatballs: Combine ingredients and form into balls. Bake in glass dish at 350 degrees for 20 minutes, turning over after 10 minutes.

Sauce: Drain pineapple; save juice and add enough water to total 1½ cups. Combine ingredients, including juice, in pot. Cook over low heat, stirring constantly until thick.

Pour sauce over meatballs and bake 10 minutes. Serve with rice.

Makes 6 servings.

Wheat Hamburger Casserole

1 cup cooked wheat
1 can corn, drained
1 finely chopped onion
1 finely chopped green pepper
1 lb. ground beef, raw and crumbled
2 cans tomato sauce
¾ cup water
grated cheese

Put wheat on the bottom of 9 x 13 pan. Layer half of corn, onion, green pepper, beef, and tomato sauce. Repeat layers. Pour water on top.

Cover and bake at 350 degrees for 1 hour. Top with grated cheese.

Makes 8 servings.

Heavenly Hash Casserole

2 lbs. ground beef
1 medium onion, finely chopped
1 stalk celery, sliced
⅛ tsp. salt
1 can cream of mushroom soup
1 can cream of chicken soup
½ cup whole wheat, cooked
½ cup water
1 can Chinese noodles

Brown meat with onion, celery, and salt. Drain grease. Add soups, wheat, and water. Cook in slow cooker on low 2–3 hours or cover and bake in oven at 350 degrees for 1 hour. Remove cover and add 1 can Chinese noodles. Bake 15 more minutes.

Makes 8 servings.

Wheat and Mushroom Veggie Casserole

1 cup water
½ pkg. dry onion soup mix
½ cup whole wheat berries
8 mushrooms, sliced thin
butter
2 scallions, sliced into rounds

Bring water and onion soup mix to a boil. Add wheat berries. Reduce heat to low and simmer until all the liquid is absorbed, about 20 minutes. Sauté mushrooms in butter. Mix mushrooms and scallions with wheat mixture. The heat of the wheat will cook the scallions.

Makes 4 servings.

Taco Casserole

This is a favorite for a busy day.

¼–½ cup cracked wheat
1 cup water
1 lb. lean ground beef
1 onion, chopped
1 pkg. taco seasoning
1 (32-oz.) can tomatoes or spaghetti sauce
1 pkg. tortillas
1 cup shredded cheese

Heat cracked wheat and water in frying pan until water is absorbed and cracked wheat is heated and half-cooked. Add ground beef and chopped onion. Sauté. Add tomatoes or spaghetti sauce and taco seasoning. Simmer. If mixture gets too thick or sticky, add water. Place a layer of tortillas in 9 x 13 pan. Layer meat mixture, shredded cheese, and tortillas. End with a top layer of shredded cheese. Bake in oven at 350 degrees for 10 minutes, or microwave 5 minutes, covered with plastic wrap.

Makes 6 servings.

Wheat Casserole

2 eggs
2 cups grated sharp cheddar cheese
2 cups cooked wheat berries
1 cup milk
¼ cup vegetable oil
1 medium onion, grated
1 tsp. salt
4 tsp. fresh parsley, chopped, or 1 tsp. dried

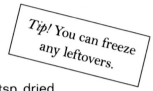

Tip! You can freeze any leftovers.

Beat eggs until thick; add grated cheese. Add wheat berries, milk, oil, onion, salt, and parsley. Mix well. Pour into 1-qt. casserole dish. Bake at 350 degrees for 1 hour. Let set 5–10 minutes.

Makes 6 servings.

Wheat Casserole Variation

1 cup wheat, soaked overnight
1 cup rice
2 pkgs. dry chicken noodle soup
6 cups water
1–2 lbs. ground beef
1 medium chopped onion
3 stalks celery, diced
1 bell pepper, diced

Bring wheat, rice, soup, and water to a boil. Simmer 45 minutes, or until wheat is tender. Brown beef with onion, celery, and pepper. Mix in to wheat mixture. Put in 1-qt. casserole dish and bake at 325 degrees for 45 minutes.

Makes 10 servings.

Broccoli Casserole

2 (10-oz.) bags chopped frozen broccoli
1 cup mayonnaise
1 can cream of mushroom soup
½ cup grated cheese
2 Tbsp. grated onion
1 cup whole wheat bread crumbs

Cook broccoli and drain. Mix with mayonnaise, soup, cheese, and onion. Put in greased casserole dish. Optional: put bread crumbs in pan with 3 tablespoons butter and toast in oven at 375 degrees until brown. Top casserole with bread crumbs. Bake at 375 degrees for 45 minutes or until crumbs are golden brown.

Makes 6 servings.

Potato Dumplings

5 medium potatoes, peeled
3 tsp. salt
1¼ cups cornstarch
½ cup hot milk
1 tsp. baking powder
1 slice stale whole wheat bread or ½ cup whole wheat croutons
butter to taste

Boil potatoes and mash or put through sieve. Add salt, cornstarch, and milk. This dough will be rather soft at first but will get firmer as it cools. When it's lukewarm, stir in baking powder. If the dough is too warm, the baking powder reacts before desired.

With floured hands, shape the dough into small balls. Press a few croutons or bread crumbs into each ball. Drop into boiling water one at a time. Simmer 20–25 minutes. Top with butter before serving.

Makes 6 servings.

Whole Wheat Veggie Pizza

Crust
2½ cups white flour
½ cup whole wheat flour
2 pkgs. quick rise yeast
1 cup lukewarm water
1 tsp. olive oil

Sauce
1 tsp. garlic powder
1 (14-oz.) can diced tomatoes
1½ tsp. sugar
2 Tbsp. olive oil
1 Tbsp. minced parsley
1½ tsp. dried basil
½ tsp. Italian seasoning

Topping
¼ tsp. hot pepper toppings
1 cup sliced fresh mushrooms
¼ cup chopped onion
¼ cup sweet red pepper
¼ cup green pepper
1 cup chopped zucchini (optional)
1¼ cup shredded mozzarella cheese

Crust: In a mixing bowl, combine flours and yeast. Add water and oil; beat until smooth. Knead on floured surface until smooth. Punch dough down and divide in half. Roll out each portion into a 12-inch circle and put on greased pizza pans. Prick with fork. Bake at 400 degrees 8–10 minutes.

Sauce: Combine ingredients in a saucepan. Bring to a boil; reduce heat. Simmer uncovered 15–18 minutes, stirring occasionally. Cool and spread lightly on crust.

Topping: In a skillet, sauté pepper toppings and vegetables until tender. Spread on pizzas and sprinkle with cheese. Bake at 400 degrees 12–15 minutes or until cheese is melted.

Salmon Loaf

Loaf
1 can salmon
1 cup whole wheat bread crumbs
¾ tsp. salt
1 cup milk
butter
3–4 hard boiled eggs, diced

White Sauce
1 Tbsp. butter
1 Tbsp. flour
1 cup milk
¼ tsp. salt
⅛ tsp. pepper

Loaf: Mix salmon, bread crumbs, salt, and milk. Place in a greased loaf pan and dot with butter. Put loaf pan on cookie sheet filled with water. Bake at 325 degrees 30–45 minutes. Let rest in pan 10 minutes.

White Sauce: Melt butter and add flour, stirring until thick. For thicker sauce, add 1 more tablespoon butter and 1 more tablespoon flour. Add milk and salt and pepper. Cook until bubbly.

Remove loaf from pan. Garnish with eggs and serve with white sauce.

Makes 8 servings.

Thin White Sauce

Delicious on vegetables!

1 Tbsp. butter
1 Tbsp. whole wheat flour
¼ tsp. salt
⅛ tsp. ground pepper
1 cup milk

Melt butter in saucepan over low heat. Add flour. Stir constantly so it doesn't burn or stick. Add salt and pepper. While stirring, gradually add milk. When it boils, it is done. It may thicken as it cools.

Makes 4 servings.

VARIATIONS (ADD AFTER SAUCE HAS BOILED)

Capers: Add 1 tablespoon drained capers and 2 tablespoons minced parsley to white sauce. Use on fish or vegetables.

Cheese: Add ½ cup diced American cheese and a dash of Worcestershire sauce. Heat gently until cheese melts. Use on cooked vegetables or pasta.

Curry: Sauté 2 tablespoons minced onion in 1 tablespoon butter. Stir in 1–2 teaspoons curry powder. Use on vegetables, eggs, fish, poultry, or other meat.

Horseradish: Stir 2 tablespoons horseradish into white sauce. Use on fish or hard cooked eggs.

Mushroom: Add ½ cup cooked sliced mushrooms to white sauce. Season with onion salt, if desired. Use on vegetables or eggs.

Mustard: Stir 2–3 tablespoons mustard into white sauce. Use on boiled beef, hard cooked eggs, or corned beef.

India Wheat Cakes

2 cups cracked wheat
½ cup chopped onion
1 tsp. baking soda
2 Tbsp. dry milk
2 eggs
½ cup fresh mint or parsley, or 1 Tbsp. dried

Mix all ingredients. Season as desired. Form into patties and fry.

Makes 6.

Boston Baked Wheat

This is similar to Boston Baked Beans.

4 cups cooked wheat
1 cup catsup
1 onion, cooked and chopped
½ cup mild molasses
3 slices bacon, cooked and crumbled
¾ tsp. mustard
1 cup water

Combine everything in baking dish and bake at 350 degrees for ½ hour. Makes 6 servings.

Tip! This tastes better the next day.

Imitation Kibbee

This is a Lebanese meatball.

Dough
1 cup fine cracked wheat
1 cup medium cracked wheat*
2 small potatoes, boiled and mashed
1 tsp. salt
pepper to taste

Tip! Try serving these in a pita.

Stuffing
½ lb. ground beef or sausage, browned
¼ lb. chopped walnuts (optional)
1 cup flour

Yogurt Sauce
1 cup plain yogurt
½ cup fresh mint, minced
salt and pepper

Dough: Mix and soak wheat in lukewarm water for 5 minutes. Wash with cold water and squeeze tightly. Place in large bowl. Add potatoes and salt and pepper. Mix well. If dough is soft, add flour 1 tablespoon at a time until dough forms into balls. Shape like footballs and make a hole in center.

Stuffing: Mix meat, walnuts, and flour. Stuff into dough's hole and cover hole. Deep fry in vegetable oil.

Yogurt Sauce: Mix yogurt, mint, and salt and pepper. Serve on top.

Makes 6 servings.

*Substitute: Use quinoa instead of cracked wheat.

Chinese Fried Wheat

1 cup cracked wheat (strain out any flour before cooking)
2½ cup water
½ tsp. salt
3 Tbsp. vegetable oil
1 egg, beaten
1 onion, minced
¼ cup celery diced
2 Tbsp. soy sauce or to taste
3 strips bacon, crumbled, or ½ cup cubed ham

Bring wheat, water, and salt to a boil. Cover and simmer 20–30 minutes. Strain to drain off thick liquid; save liquid for gravy. Wash wheat with cold water to make fluffy. Press wheat with paper towel to remove all moisture possible and set aside.

Heat 1 tablespoon oil in heavy skillet. Slowly add egg, stirring rapidly with fork so egg is light and fluffy. Set aside.

In skillet, add 2 tablespoons of oil, onion, and celery; cook until tender. Add wheat, soy sauce, bacon or ham, and egg. Heat.

Serve with rice and Chinese noodles.

Makes 6 servings.

Gluten

Gluten is the protein part of the wheat. It is listed as a principal source of protein, the same as eggs, meat, fish, milk, cheese, soybeans, tofu, and peanuts. Protein is important in sustaining life. The body uses protein to repair its cells. The proteins must constantly be replaced because the body does not store protein.

In wheat, gluten holds the carbon dioxide that is made from yeast, enabling dough to rise. Gluten contains two principal proteins, glutenin and gliadin. Gliadin allows the gluten to be elastic after it eliminates the starch and bran.

After wheat is ground into flour, gluten can be separated from the other parts of the flour by adding water until it's very thick, mixing, kneading, and pounding while washing the mixture in a bowl of water. The more the mixture is washed, the more elastic it will become, similar to candy taffy. The amount of gluten depends on the protein content of the wheat. A hard winter wheat gets the best results.

The amount needed is determined by the person's age and weight.

Conversion
7 cups whole wheat flour yields 1–2 cups of raw gluten
1 cup raw gluten = 72 grams protein
1 oz. ground beef = 6 grams protein

Never use a 100 percent whole wheat diet. Gluten builds up on the intestinal walls and prohibits the absorption of glucose and other nutrients, causing malnourishment.

References

Moulton, Le Arta. *The Gluten Book.* Provo, Utah: The Gluten Co., 1977.

Robertson, Laurel, Carol Flinders, and Bronwen Godfrey. *Laurel's Kitchen Bread Book.* Berkeley, California: Niligri Press, 1976.

Tyler, Lorranine Dilwort. *The Magic of Wheat Cookery.* Provo, Utah: Community Press, 1977.

Gluten Patties in Mushroom Sauce

½ cup soy sauce
⅛ tsp. garlic salt
½ tsp. sage
2 eggs
1 medium onion, chopped
2 cups cooked rice
2 cups gluten, ground
1 can mushroom soup

Mix soy sauce, garlic salt, sage, eggs, and onion together. Add rice and gluten. Shape into patties. Fry slowly in vegetable oil until browned. Add mushroom soup with ¼ cup water, simmering 10–15 minutes.

Makes 6 servings.

Gluten Sausage

1 cup ground gluten
1 lb. ground sausage
1 Tbsp. flour
1 egg
½ cup butter or margarine

Combine gluten and sausage. Flavor with any choice of seasonings. Mix in flour and egg. Form into patties. Fry in butter or margarine, browning on both sides.

Makes 4 servings.

Gluten Burger

2–3 Tbsp. beef base
2 cups ground gluten
1 egg
1 medium onion, finely chopped
salt and pepper to taste
whole wheat flour
½ cup butter or margarine

Combine beef base and gluten. Stir in egg, onion, and salt and pepper. Add enough flour to make patties. Fry in butter or margarine, browning both sides. Steam in covered saucepan 5 minutes.

Makes 4 servings.

Beef Substitute

Use this as a substitute to ground beef.

2 cups gluten
3 Tbsp. beef base to taste

Simmer gluten and beef flavoring. Grind with meat grinder. Substitute full amount or use ½ substitute and ½ ground beef.

Cookies

Whole Wheat Cookies

½ cup vegetable oil
½ cup brown sugar
½ cup honey
2 eggs
1 tsp. vanilla
2 cups whole wheat flour
1 tsp. baking soda
½ tsp. salt
½ cup milk
1 cup chopped nuts (optional)
1 cup raisins (optional)

Cream oil, sugar, and honey. Gradually beat in eggs and vanilla. In another bowl, sift flour, baking soda, and salt. Gradually add flour mixture and milk to sugar mixture; mix well. Add nuts and raisins, if desired. Drop by spoonful onto greased baking sheet. Bake at 350 degrees 10–12 minutes.

Makes 2 dozen.

Whole Wheat Orange Cookies

1 cup sugar
1 tsp. baking powder
½ tsp. salt
½ tsp. baking soda
1 tsp. vanilla
½ tsp. nutmeg
½ cup margarine
2 Tbsp. milk
2 Tbsp. grated orange peel
1 egg
2 cups whole wheat flour

Combine all ingredients except the whole wheat flour. Add flour and roll into 1-inch balls. Roll in cinnamon-sugar blend (mix ½ cup sugar with 2 teaspoons cinnamon). Bake on cookie sheet at 375 degrees 8–10 minutes.

Makes 2 dozen.

Whole Wheat Chocolate Chip Cookies

1½ cups brown sugar
1 cup butter, softened
1 tsp. vanilla
3 eggs
2½ cups whole wheat flour
⅓ cup dry milk powder
1 tsp. baking soda
½ tsp. salt
¾ cup chopped pecans
2 cups chocolate chips
½ cup sunflower seeds

Preheat oven to 350 degrees. In large bowl, cream brown sugar, butter, vanilla, and eggs. Stir in flour, dry milk, baking soda, and salt. Stir in pecans, chocolate chips, and sunflower seeds. Drop by spoonful 2 inches apart onto greased cookie sheets. Bake 10–14 minutes or until light brown.

Makes 5–6 dozen.

Whole Wheat Walnut Chocolate Chip Cookies

1 cup unsalted butter, at room temperature
1½ cups brown sugar
2 eggs
1 tsp. vanilla
2 cups whole wheat flour
¼ cup quick oatmeal
1 tsp. baking soda
½ tsp. salt
1¼ cups semisweet chocolate chips
1 cup chopped walnuts

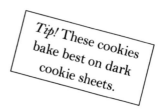

Tip! These cookies bake best on dark cookie sheets.

Preheat oven to 350 degrees. In medium bowl, beat butter with electric mixer until soft. Add brown sugar and beat until light and fluffy. Beat in vanilla and eggs one at a time. In a separate bowl, stir together flour, oatmeal, baking soda, and salt. Add gradually to batter, stirring just until blended. Stir in chocolate chips and walnuts. Use a spoon to drop pieces of dough slightly smaller than a golf ball onto baking sheets, leaving about 3 inches between pieces. Bake one sheet at a time 12–14 minutes. Cookies have slightly uneven, golden brown coloring. They may seem undercooked in the middle, but will firm up. Let cool on sheet several minutes, and then transfer to wire rack. Cool thoroughly before storing in airtight container.

Makes 3 dozen.

Whole Wheat Honey Butter Cookies

1 cup unsalted butter, softened
⅔ cup honey
2 large eggs
½ tsp. vanilla
2⅓ cups whole wheat flour
1 tsp. baking powder
½ tsp. salt
½ tsp. cinnamon

Preheat oven to 375 degrees. Beat butter and honey with an electric mixer until soft and creamy. Beat in eggs one at a time. Stir in vanilla. Into a separate bowl, sift whole wheat flour with baking powder, salt, and cinnamon. Add gradually to batter, stirring just until blended. Cover dough and refrigerate 30 minutes. Using floured hands, make balls of dough about 1¼ inches in diameter. (If desired, roll them in additional sugar or a cinnamon-sugar blend—½ cup sugar with 2 teaspoons cinnamon). You can leave balls rounded or flatten them a little with the tines of a fork. Bake one sheet at a time for 10 minutes. Cool cookies on sheet, then transfer to wire rack to cool. Store in airtight container.

Makes 2 dozen.

Whole Wheat Peanut Butter Cookies

½ cup butter or margarine, softened
½ cup peanut butter
½ cup sugar
½ cup brown sugar
1 egg
½ tsp. vanilla
1¼ cups whole wheat flour
½ tsp. baking powder
¾ tsp. baking soda
¼ tsp. salt

Cream together butter, peanut butter, sugar, brown sugar, egg, and vanilla until light and fluffy. In a separate bowl, combine flour, baking powder, baking soda, and salt, blending well. Stir into creamed mixture. Cover dough and refrigerate several hours or overnight. Shape dough into balls about ¾-inch in diameter. Place balls 3 inches apart on a greased cookie sheet; flatten each cookie with the tines of a fork. Bake at 375 degrees 8–12 minutes or until set, but not hard.

Makes 4 dozen.

Applesauce Cookies

2 cups whole wheat flour
1 tsp. baking powder
½ tsp. salt
½ tsp. baking soda
½ tsp. ground cloves
1 tsp. cinnamon
½ cup butter
1 cup brown sugar
2 eggs
½ tsp. vanilla
½–1 cup thick applesauce
1 cup raisins
1 cup chopped nuts (optional)

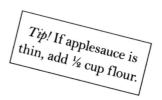

Tip! If applesauce is thin, add ½ cup flour.

Sift flour two times; add baking powder, salt, baking soda, ground cloves, and cinnamon. Cream butter and brown sugar; add eggs and beat well. Add vanilla and applesauce. Add raisins and nuts. Drop by spoonful on greased cookie sheet. Bake at 350 degrees 10–12 minutes.

Makes 3 dozen.

German Whole Grain Crumb Cookies

1½ cups fine whole wheat bread crumbs*
1½ cups finely chopped walnuts
⅔ cup brown sugar
⅓ cup granulated sugar
½ tsp. cinnamon
½ tsp. ground cloves
½ tsp. nutmeg
¼ tsp. cardamom
¼ tsp. salt
6 Tbsp. butter cut in pieces
1 large egg, lightly beaten
¼ cup unbleached flour

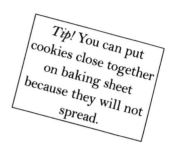

Tip! You can put cookies close together on baking sheet because they will not spread.

In a large bowl, mix bread crumbs, walnuts, brown and granulated sugar, cinnamon, cloves, nutmeg, cardamom, and salt. Rub them together with your hands until smooth—this brings out the flavor. Add butter and rub in until mixture has coarse, uniform texture. Drizzle egg over top and work in with hands until mixture is damp and gravelly. Work in flour.

Drop by spoonful on greased cookie sheet. Bake at 350 degrees until surface of cookies feels mostly firm to touch, about 15 minutes. Cool cookies on sheet 5 minutes, then transfer to wire rack. Store in airtight container.

*Bread crumbs: Grate dry slices of whole wheat bread using the big holes of a box grater. You will need 1½ cups to layer about ¼-inch deep in 9 x 13 baking pan. Bake at 300 degrees for 30 minutes, stirring every 10 minutes. When crumbs feel dry, remove from oven and cool in pan. Blend crumbs until very fine.

Makes 3 dozen.

Desserts

Popped Wheat Treats

These morsels are great on salads, in trail mix, on desserts, or as a snack on their own.

1½ cups whole wheat berries
vegetable oil

Boil whole wheat until kernels are plump and tender; some may begin to split. Drain and rinse. Remove excess water by rolling wheat on a cloth or paper towel. In a heavy kettle or deep fat fryer, heat oil to 360 degrees. Put wheat in wire basket or strainer and deep fry for 1½ minutes or until popping ceases. Wheat will not always pop and may be more nut-like. Drain on absorbent paper, such as paper grocery bags.

VARIATIONS
Salty: Season with salt, seasoned salt, garlic salt, barbecue salt, onion salt, or celery salt.
Sweet: Season with 2 parts cinnamon and 4 parts sugar.

Whole Wheat Candy

3 Tbsp. cocoa
½ cup milk
2 cups sugar
¼ tsp. salt
1 tsp. vanilla
1 cup cooked wheat
2 cups quick-cooking oatmeal
½ cup shredded coconut

Combine cocoa, milk, sugar, salt, and vanilla and bring to a boil. Remove from heat and add wheat, oatmeal, and coconut. Drop on waxed paper by spoonfuls. Put in refrigerator to set.

Makes 30 pieces.

Wheat Sprout Candy

1 cup wheat sprouts
1 cup raisins, dates, or figs (each or in combination)
1 cup chopped nuts
1 cup coconut

Set aside coconut and mix other ingredients. Shape into small balls and roll in coconut. Store in refrigerator.

Makes 2½ dozen.

Sprouted Wheat Nut Drops

2 cups sprouted wheat
1 cup chopped nuts
1¼ cups bread crumbs
¼ cup milk powder
3 Tbsp. powdered sugar
1 tsp. salt
1 sweet onion, minced (optional)

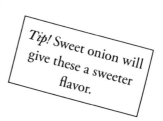

Tip! Sweet onion will give these a sweeter flavor.

Grind wheat sprouts. Mix in other ingredients. Shape into small balls and place on slightly greased baking sheet. Bake at 400 degrees 15–30 minutes, depending on size. They should be crisp and cooked in the middle.

Optional: Top with buttercream icing to serve (recipe on p. 91).

Prize-Winning Brownies

¼ cup butter
1 cup brown sugar
1 tsp. vanilla
1 egg
2 squares baking chocolate, melted
1 cup whole wheat flour
¼ tsp. salt
1 tsp. baking powder
½ can evaporated milk
1 cup chopped nuts

Cream together butter, brown sugar, and vanilla. Add egg and beat until light and fluffy. Add melted chocolate, flour, salt, and baking powder, and milk. Mix well. Pour into buttered 9 x 9 pan. Bake at 350 degrees 30–35 minutes. Cool before cutting.

Rich Chocolate Whole Wheat Brownies

2 cups sugar
½ cup margarine
4 eggs, beaten
4 squares baking chocolate, melted
⅓ cup whole wheat flour
1 cup white flour
1 cup milk
1 cup chopped nuts
1 tsp. almond flavoring
2 tsp. vanilla

Cream sugar, margarine, and eggs. Add melted chocolate. Stir in flours. Add milk and stir until smooth. Add nuts, almond flavoring, and vanilla. Bake in greased 9 x 13 pan at 375 degrees for 20 minutes. Let cool before cutting.

Makes 8 servings.

Whole Wheat Brownies

2½ cup brown sugar
½ cup butter
4 eggs
¾ cup whole wheat flour
¾ cup white flour
1 tsp. baking powder
½ cup cocoa powder
1 tsp. salt
1 Tbsp. vanilla
1 cup milk
¼ cup water

Cream brown sugar and butter. Add eggs, stirring well. Blend in dry ingredients, alternating with vanilla, milk, and water. Mix well to smooth batter. Bake in a 9 x 13 pan at 350 degrees for 45 minutes.

Makes 8 servings.

Spoon Cake

½ cup brown sugar
1 Tbsp. orange juice concentrate*
½ cup cream
2 eggs, beaten
¼ tsp. salt
¼ tsp. baking soda
1½ tsp. baking powder
1½ tsp. cinnamon
1½ cups cooked and pureed soybeans

Mix all ingredients but soybeans. Slowly beat soybeans into ingredients. Pour into greased 9 x 9 cake pan. Bake at 350 degrees for 30 minutes. Frost if desired (see buttercream icing recipe on p. 91).

*Substitute: 1 teaspoon lemonade concentrate.

Whole Wheat Spice Cake

1 cup boiling water
1 cup quick-cooking oatmeal
½ cup butter or margarine, softened
1 cup honey
2 eggs, beaten
¼ cup quick-cooking oatmeal
1 cup whole wheat flour
½ cup flour
2 tsp. baking powder
½ tsp. salt
½ tsp. ground cloves
2 tsp. ground cinnamon
¼ cup sesame seeds
¾ cup raisins
1 cup chopped dates

Topping
1 (14-oz.) can sweetened condensed milk
1 (6-oz.) pkg. semisweet chocolate chips
1 cup chopped pecans

Combine 1 cup boiling water and 1 cup oatmeal; set aside for 25 minutes. Cream butter and honey until smooth; add eggs and ¼ cup oatmeal, mixing well. Stir in flours, baking powder, salt, cloves, cinnamon, oatmeal, sesame seeds, raisins, and dates. Pour mixture into a greased 9 x 13 pan. Bake at 350 degrees for 35 minutes or until sides separate from pan.

Topping: Combine condensed milk, chocolate chips, and pecans; spread over hot cake. Return to oven for 8 minutes. Let cool.

Makes 15 servings.

Oatmeal Mush Cake

1¼ cups boiling water
1 Tbsp. butter
1 cup oatmeal
1 cup brown sugar
1 cup white sugar
2 eggs
1⅓ cups whole wheat flour
1 tsp. baking soda
1 tsp. cinnamon
½ tsp. nutmeg
½ tsp. salt

Topping
1 cup nuts chopped
1 cup coconut
6 Tbsp. margarine
½ cup sugar
1 tsp. vanilla
¼ cup canned milk

Soak butter and oatmeal in water for 20 minutes. Cream brown sugar, white sugar, and eggs. Add oatmeal mixture. Add whole wheat flour, baking soda, cinnamon, nutmeg, and salt. Stir and mix well. Pour into 8 x 8 pan. Bake at 350 degrees for 50 minutes.

Topping: Combine ingredients and mix well. Sprinkle on hot cake and bake at 400 degrees for 7 minutes, or until topping is bubbly.

Makes 8 servings.

Hot Fudge Cake

Don't hassle with dishes—mix and bake in one dish!

1¾ cups brown sugar
1 cup flour
¼ cup plus 3 Tbsp. unsweetened cocoa
2 tsp. baking powder
½ tsp. salt
½ cup milk
2 Tbsp. margarine
½ tsp. vanilla
1¾ cups boiling water
¾ cup brown sugar
¼ cup unsweetened cocoa

Mix brown sugar, flour, cocoa, baking powder, and salt in 1½-qt. pan or slow cooker. Stir in milk, margarine, and vanilla. Sprinkle brown sugar and cocoa over the top—do not stir. Pour boiling water over top and do not stir. Cook 1½–2 hours on low or 3 hours on high in slow cooker.

Chocolate Vinegar Cake

Vinegar helps the cake rise and be fluffy!

2 cups white flour
1 cup whole wheat flour
1 tsp. salt
⅔ cup cocoa
¾ cup vegetable oil
2 Tbsp. vinegar
2 tsp. baking soda
2 tsp. vanilla
2 cups water

Mix flours, salt, and cocoa. Put mixture in greased 9 x 13 pan. Make 3 holes in cake. In the first hole, put vegetable oil. In the second, put vinegar and baking soda. In the third, put vanilla. Pour water over cake and stir well. Bake at 350 degrees for 40 minutes. Frost if desired (recipe below).

Makes 8 servings.

Buttercream Icing

3 cups powdered sugar
½ cup margarine
1½ tsp. vanilla
2 Tbsp. milk

Mix sugar and margarine till blended smooth. Stir in vanilla then drip in milk slowly until you get the right consistency.

Boiled Raisin Cake

This is also called Poor Man's Cake because it doesn't use eggs or milk. It was used during the Great Depression.

2 cups water
2 cups raisins
1½ cups sugar
2 heaping Tbsp. shortening
1½ cups white flour
1½ cups whole wheat flour
1 tsp. baking soda
½ tsp. salt
1 tsp. cinnamon
¼ tsp. ground cloves
½ tsp. nutmeg
1 cup chopped nuts (optional)

Boil raisins, sugar, and shortening in water. Let cool. Mix with the rest of the ingredients. Bake in greased 9 x 13 pan at 350 degrees 35–40 minutes.

Makes 10 servings.

Applesauce Cake

Cake

1½ cups pureed soybeans
1 cup brown sugar
½ cup vegetable oil
4 eggs, beaten
¾ cup applesauce
2 cups milk
2 cups whole wheat flour
4 tsp. baking powder
1 tsp. salt
2½ tsp. cinnamon
1½ cups raisins

Glaze

½ cup honey
1 Tbsp. water
2 Tbsp. lemon peel (lemon zest)

Cake: Cream soybeans, brown sugar, and oil. Add eggs, applesauce, and milk. Mix well. Mix dry ingredients together, then add to soybean mixture. Add raisins. Put in greased 9 x 13 pan. Bake at 350 degrees for 40 minutes.

Glaze: Mix ingredients. Puncture holes in cake with fork and drizzle glaze over hot cake.

Mock Apple Pie

pie crust pastry for top and bottom
15 soda or Ritz crackers
1 cup water
1½ cups sugar
1½ tsp. cream of tartar
¼ tsp. cinnamon
¼ tsp. nutmeg
butter

Line a pie plate with pastry. Break crackers into quarters and arrange in the crust. Boil water, sugar, cream of tartar, cinnamon, and nutmeg. Pour over crackers in the crust. Add dots of butter. Cover with crust and bake at 350 degrees until brown.

Makes 6 servings.

Soybean Pie

This is like pumpkin pie.

1½ cups cooked and pureed soybeans
1⅔ cups milk
¾ cup evaporated milk
1 cup brown sugar
3 tsp. grated lemon
½ cup vanilla
1½ tsp. cinnamon
1¼ tsp. ginger
¾ tsp. ground cloves
½ tsp. nutmeg
2 eggs, beaten
unbaked pie shell

Combine soybeans and milks in blender or mixer. Blend in remaining ingredients. Pour into unbaked pie shell. Bake at 400 degrees 40–50 minutes, or until a knife comes out clean. Serve with ice cream or whipped cream.

Crunchy Wheat Pie Crust

1⅓ cups fine wheat crumbs from bread or cereal
¼ cup melted margarine

Combine bread crumbs and margarine. Press into 8-inch pie tin.

To use: Pour pie filling into the shell and refrigerate until firmly set.

Whole Wheat Pie Crust

1 cup plus 2 Tbsp. whole wheat flour
1 Tbsp. sugar
⅛ tsp. salt
7 Tbsp. vegetable oil
2 Tbsp. cold water

Blend ingredients in bowl. Press into 9-inch pie tin.

To use: Bake as directed for pie recipe.

Lemon Cream Pie

1 cup water
⅛ tsp. salt
½ cup water
⅓ cup wheat flour
⅓ cup dry milk powder
⅔ cup sugar
½ cup cold water
1 tsp. gelatin (⅓ of envelope)
2 Tbsp. cold water
1 pkg. sugar-free lemonade powder

Boil 1 cup water and salt. Make a paste with ½ cup water and flour. Slowly pour mixture into boiling water, stirring constantly. Let cook on low heat 7–8 minutes, stirring frequently. Remove from heat. In small mixing bowl, combine dry milk powder, sugar, and ½ cup cold water. Set aside. Soften gelatin in 2 tablespoons cold water, put on low heat, and stir until dissolved. Add to milk mixture and stir until thickened. Add lemonade powder. Mix until dissolved. Combine with cooked wheat and mix well. Pour into 8-inch pie crust and serve with whipped topping.

Coconut Cream Pie

1 Tbsp. cracked wheat
¼ tsp. coconut flavoring or to taste

Make lemon cream pie filling, except replace lemonade powder with cracked wheat soaked in coconut flavoring. Add coconut flavoring when all ingredients are mixed together.

Chocolate Cream Pie

1 Tbsp. cocoa
½ tsp. vanilla

Make lemon cream pie, except add cocoa and vanilla instead of lemonade powder.

Poor Man's Pudding

Don't hassle with dishes—mix and bake in one dish!

½ cup white flour
½ cup whole wheat flour
2 tsp. baking powder
¼ tsp. salt
½ cup sugar
½ tsp. nutmeg
½ cup raisins
½ cup milk
1¾ cups boiling water
2 Tbsp. butter or margarine
¾ cup brown sugar
½ tsp. vanilla

Mix flours, baking powder, salt, sugar, nutmeg, and raisins in 8 x 8 dish. Add milk. Boil water, butter, and brown sugar. Remove from heat and add vanilla. Pour over flour mixture—do not stir. Bake at 350 degrees 40–50 minutes. Serve warm with whipped topping.

Makes 6 servings.

Bread Pudding

Pudding
4 cups stale whole wheat bread
¼ cup chopped nuts
3 Tbsp. raisins
3 eggs
8 Tbsp. sugar
3 cups milk
1 tsp. vanilla

Topping
2 slices whole wheat bread, broken into crumbs
3 Tbsp. brown sugar
2 Tbsp. butter

Pudding: Cut bread in ¾-inch squares and fill a 1-qt. baking dish to within ½-inch from the top. Mix in nuts and raisins. In a bowl, whip eggs. Add sugar, milk, and vanilla. Pour over bread. Do not mix.

Topping: Work brown sugar and butter into crumbs and sprinkle over pudding. Bake at 375 degrees for 1 hour. Cool and serve.

Makes 8 servings.

Nutty Apple and Wheat Betty

2½ cups cooked wheat
3 Tbsp. peanut butter
1½ Tbsp. sugar
¼ tsp. cinnamon
½ tsp. vanilla
1 can apple pie filling*
1 tsp. lemon juice
⅛ tsp. nutmeg

Blend wheat, peanut butter, sugar, cinnamon, and vanilla in medium bowl. Combine apple pie filling and wheat mixture alternately in greased 9 x 9 dish. Sprinkle lemon juice and nutmeg on top. Bake at 350 degrees 20–25 minutes.

*Substitute: Mix 1½ cups sliced apples, ¼ cup brown sugar, ½ cup sugar, and 2 tablespoons flour; increase cinnamon to ½ teaspoon.

Makes 6–8 servings.

Banana Wheat Custard

1 Tbsp. butter
⅓ cup sugar
½ cup mashed banana
2 eggs, slightly beaten
2 cups milk
1 Tbsp. lemon juice
1 tsp. grated lemon rind
1 tsp. vanilla
⅛ tsp. salt
1½ cups cooked wheat

Cream butter, sugar, and banana. Blend in eggs and milk. Add lemon juice and rind, vanilla, and salt. Slowly add wheat until well mixed. Place in 8 x 8 baking dish. Place baking dish in pan of water. Water should come no more than halfway up the baking dish. Bake at 350 degrees 40–50 minutes.

Makes 6 servings.

Summer Crisp

½ cup sugar
3 Tbsp. flour
1 tsp. grated lemon peel
¾ tsp. lemon juice
4 cups peaches, freshly sliced or canned and drained
3 cups blueberries, fresh or thawed

Topping
⅔ cup quick-cooking oatmeal
⅓ cup brown sugar
⅓ cup whole wheat flour
2 tsp. ground cinnamon
1 Tbsp. soft margarine

Combine sugar, flour, and lemon peel. Stir in lemon juice and fruit. Spoon into 1½-qt. baking dish.

Topping: Combine oatmeal, brown sugar, flour, and cinnamon. Stir in melted margarine. Sprinkle topping over filling. Bake at 375 degrees 40–50 minutes or until filling is bubbly and top is brown. Serve warm.

Makes 8 servings.

Mixes and Substitutes

All-Purpose Mix

5 lbs. white flour
5 cups dry milk powder
½ cup sugar
¾ cup baking powder
3 Tbsp. salt
2 Tbsp. cream of tartar
2 lbs. shortening

Sift flour, dry milk, sugar, baking powder, salt, and cream of tartar. Cut in shortening until mixture looks like cornmeal. Store in gallon jars or large containers with tight lids at room temperature until used.

Makes 1½ gallons.

Gingerbread

1 egg
½ cup water
½ cup molasses
2 cups all-purpose mix
¼ cup sugar
½ tsp. cinnamon
½ tsp. ginger
½ tsp. cloves

Beat egg; add water and molasses. Blend well. Blend all-purpose mix with sugar and spices. Gradually combine all ingredients and mix well. Pour in greased 8 x 8 pan. Bake at 350 degrees for 40 minutes.

Makes 6 servings.

Dutch Apple Cake

2 cups all-purpose mix
1 tsp. cinnamon
¾ cup plus 2 Tbsp. sugar
1 egg
⅔ cup water
½ tsp. vanilla
2 cups cooking apples, peeled and sliced
cinnamon-sugar blend (½ cup sugar and 2 tsp. cinnamon)
¼ cup melted butter

Mix all-purpose mix, cinnamon, and sugar. In a separate bowl, beat egg; add water and vanilla. Gradually add to dry ingredients. Stir until batter is smooth. Pour into a greased 8 x 8 pan. Place apples slices in rows on top. Sprinkle with cinnamon-sugar blend and pour melted butter over top. Bake at 375 degrees for 30 minutes. Serve warm with whipped cream or lemon sauce (recipe below).

Makes 6 servings.

Lemon Sauce

1 Tbsp. cornstarch
½ cup sugar
pinch of salt
1 cup boiling water
1 Tbsp. butter
grated rind of ½ lemon
¼ cup lemon juice

Boil cornstarch, sugar, salt, and water. Stir in butter, rind, and lemon juice; stir gently until desired consistency.

Orange Bread

1 cup water
½ cup grated orange rind (orange zest)
1 egg
1 cup orange juice
½ cup sugar
3 cups all-purpose mix
½ cup chopped nuts

Boil water and orange zest. Cook 5 minutes. Strain, discarding liquid. In medium bowl, beat egg and add orange juice. Add sugar and all-purpose mix. Stir to blend, but do not overmix. Add orange zest and nuts. Pour into greased loaf pan. Bake at 375 degrees for 35 minutes.

Oatmeal Cookies

3 cups all-purpose mix
1 cup sugar
1 cup quick-cooking oatmeal
1 tsp. cinnamon
1 egg
⅓ cup water
½ cup chopped nuts (optional)

Stir together mix, sugar, oatmeal, and cinnamon. Beat egg with water. Stir into dry ingredients. Add nuts if desired. Mix will be stiff. Drop on greased cookie sheet. Bake at 400 degrees 10–12 minutes.

Makes 4 dozen.

Banana Bread

3 cups all-purpose mix
½ cup sugar
1½ cups mashed bananas
1 egg
¼ cup water
½ cup chopped nuts (optional)

Blend all-purpose mix and sugar. In separate bowl, blend mashed bananas, egg, and water. Mix with dry ingredients; do not overbeat. Add nuts and pour into a greased loaf pan. Bake at 400 degrees for 30 minutes.

All-Purpose Applesauce Cake

3 cups all-purpose mix
1 cup sugar
½ tsp. cinnamon
½ tsp. allspice
2 eggs
½ cup water
2 Tbsp. vegetable oil
1½ cups canned applesauce

Blend all-purpose mix, sugar, and spices. In a separate bowl, beat eggs; add water, oil, and applesauce. Add half of this to dry ingredients and blend well. Add remaining liquid and mix well. Pour into two greased 8 x 8 pans and bake at 375 degrees for 30 minutes. Let cool. Frost if desired (see buttercream icing on p. 91 or glaze on p. 93).

Chocolate Devil Cake

3 cups all-purpose mix
1½ cups sugar
½ cup cocoa
1 cup water
2 eggs
2 Tbsp. oil
1 tsp. vanilla
¼ tsp. red food coloring (optional)

Mix dry ingredients. Add wet ingredients and mix well. Add red food coloring, if desired. Pour into 2 greased 8 x 8 pans. Bake at 350 degrees for 35 minutes. Cool and frost.

Coffee Cake

Cake
1 egg
⅔ cup water
⅓ cup sugar
3 cups all-purpose mix

Topping
⅓ cup butter or margarine
1 tsp. cinnamon
1 cup brown sugar

Cake: Beat egg and add water. In a separate bowl, blend sugar and all-purpose mix. Stir in liquid. Pour into greased 8 x 8 pan.

Topping: Blend butter, cinnamon, and brown sugar until well mixed. Cover cake batter evenly. Bake at 400 degrees for 25 minutes.

Makes 8 servings.

Pancakes or Waffles

1 egg
1½ cups water
3 cups all-purpose mix

Beat egg and add water. Pour half of the liquid into the mix and blend. Add remaining liquid and mix until blended. Pour onto greased hot griddle or into hot waffle iron.

Makes 12 pancakes or 6 waffles.

VARIATION: Add ¾ cup drained blueberries or ½ cup chopped nuts to batter.

Deluxe Pancakes

2 cups all-purpose mix
⅔ cup water
3 eggs
creamed chicken, turkey, or tuna*
sharp cheddar cheese, grated

Mix all-purpose mix, water, and eggs. Bake on griddle for pancakes. Fill with creamed chicken, turkey, or tuna and roll up like a burrito. Fasten with toothpick. Sprinkle with cheese and put in oven or microwave to heat through and melt cheese.

*Creamed chicken, turkey, or tuna: Make a basic white sauce and add ¼ cup cubed meat. Or use cream of mushroom soup with ¼ cup water. Mix well and add ¼ cup of meat.

Cake Mix

8 cups white flour
5 cups sugar
¼ cup baking powder
4 tsp. salt
2 cups shortening

Mix dry ingredients thoroughly. Drop shortening by spoonfuls onto dry ingredients. Blend and cut in with pastry blender until mix is the consistency of cornmeal, scraping bowl frequently. Store in four ziplock plastic bags of 3½ cups at room temperature. Do not refrigerate. Keeps several months in cool, dark place. To measure, spoon lightly into measuring cup.

Makes 14 cups, enough for four cakes.

Orange or Lemon Cake

3½ cups cake mix
1 tsp. grated orange peel (orange zest)*
¼ cup milk
2 Tbsp. orange juice*

Mix cake mix and orange zest. Add milk and orange juice and beat 2 minutes. Pour into 2 greased and floured 8-inch round pans. Bake at 350 degrees 25–30 minutes. Cool 10 minutes and remove from pan.

Makes 10 servings.

*For lemon cake, use lemon peel and lemon juice instead of orange. Add 2 tablespoons of sugar if desired.

Banana Cake

3½ cups cake mix
1 tsp. baking soda
½ cup milk
2 eggs
1 cup mashed ripe banana
½ cup chopped nuts

Combine cake mix and baking soda. Add milk, eggs, and banana; beat until well mixed. Fold in nuts. Pour into 2 greased and floured 8 x 8 cake or loaf pans. Bake at 350 degrees 25–30 minutes.

Cool 10 minutes in pans. Remove from pans and cool on racks.

Makes 8 servings.

Corn Bread Mix

8 cups cornmeal
2 cups flour
4 Tbsp. baking powder
4 tsp. salt
1 Tbsp. sugar
2²/₃ cups dry milk powder
1 cup vegetable oil

Sift together cornmeal, flour, baking powder, salt, sugar, and dry milk powder in large bowl. Pour oil over entire surface and blend in with a large spoon. Store in a covered jar at room temperature.

Makes 3 quarts.

Oven Corn Bread

2 eggs
1 cup water
2 cups corn bread mix

Beat eggs, add water. Pour half over mix and stir to blend. Add rest of liquid and beat until batter is smooth. Pour in greased 8 x 8 pan and bake at 400 degrees 20–25 minutes.

Makes 4–6 servings.

Corn Bread Muffins

2 cups corn bread mix
1 Tbsp. sugar
2 eggs
1 cup water
1 Tbsp. oil

Blend corn bread mix and sugar. In a separate bowl, beat egg; add water and oil. Pour half of liquid into mix. Blend. Add rest of liquid and blend. Fill greased muffin tins ⅔ full. Bake at 400 degrees for 20 minutes.

Makes 1 dozen.

All-Purpose Biscuits

3 cups all-purpose mix
⅔ cup water

Stir all-purpose mix and water until mix is wet and blended. Put on floured surface. Knead lightly 10 strokes—do not overknead. Roll out ¼-inch thick and cut with cookie cutter or round drinking glass, or shape with hands. Bake on greased cookie sheet at 450 degrees for 10 minutes.

Makes 12 large or 18 medium biscuits.

VARIATIONS

Bread Sticks: Roll out dough. Cut into strips 3 x ½ inch. Grease baking sheet generously with 2 tablespoons melted butter. Baking pan may be greased with garlic butter for garlic sticks. Lay strips into pan not quite touching. Brush tops with melted butter and sprinkle with caraway, sesame or poppy seeds, or other mixed dried herbs. Bake at 425 degrees for 10 minutes. Serve hot.

Cheese: Add ½ cup grated sharp cheese to mix before adding water.

Cinnamon Rolls: Roll out dough into a rectangle. Sprinkle with ⅓ cup sugar mixed with 1 teaspoon cinnamon. Dot with butter. Roll up like a jelly roll. Slice and put in greased muffin tins. Bake at 425 degrees 15–20 minutes. Icing: Mix ½ cup powdered sugar with 2 tablespoons cream or milk. It should be stiff. Ice while rolls are hot.

Cobbler Topping: Make biscuits. Roll dough out ⅛-inch thick. Place dough on cobbler mix in pan. Trim edge and cut holes in top. Brush with melted butter and sprinkle with sugar. Bake at 400 degrees for 20 minutes.

Fruit Shortcake: Beat an egg, add ½ cup water and 3 cups all-purpose mix. Roll out ¼-inch thin and cut with cookie cutter. Place two biscuits together with a slice of butter between. Bake at 425 degrees for 15 minutes. Put fruit of your choice between 2 biscuits and top with whipped cream or topping. Makes 8 servings.

Four-Grain Griddle Cake Mix

3 cups whole wheat flour
1 cup oatmeal
1 cup soybean flour
1 cup flour made from popcorn (grind popcorn in blender)
2 tsp. salt
½ cup sugar (optional)
4 Tbsp. baking powder
½ cup shortening

Mix dry ingredients together evenly. Cut in the shortening by hand to make even throughout the mixture.

Griddle Cakes

1 egg
¾ cup water
¼ cup oil
1 cup griddle cake mix

Mix ingredients until smooth and bake on hot greased griddle.

Biscuit Mix

3 cups flour
¼ cup baking powder
1 Tbsp. salt
2 Tbsp. sugar
2 cups dry powdered milk
1½ cups shortening

Sift dry ingredients. Cut in shortening until mixture has a fine, even crumb texture. Cover tightly and store in refrigerator. Will last up to six months in a cool, dry place.

Makes 1½ quarts.

Biscuits

2 cups biscuit mix
½ cup milk

Blend in bowl. Knead on floured surface gently one minute. Pat or roll to ½-inch thick and cut with biscuit cutter. Bake at 450 degrees 12–15 minutes.

Makes 10–12 biscuits.

VARIATIONS

Blueberry Muffins: Mix 5 cups biscuit mix, 1 cup sugar, 3 slightly beaten eggs, 4 tablespoons melted butter, 1 can blueberries drained, and 1½ cups milk. Spoon into muffin pans. Bake at 400 degrees 15–18 minutes.

Bran Muffins: Mix 4 cups biscuit mix, 1 cup all bran, 1 cup sugar, 3 slightly beaten eggs, 4 tablespoons melted butter, and 1½ cup milk. Spoon into muffin pans. Bake at 400 degrees for 15–18 minutes.

Breakfast Cake: Mix 2 cups biscuit mix, 2 tablespoons sugar, and 1 egg, thoroughly. Bake at 400 degrees for 30 minutes.

Dumplings: Mix 2 cups biscuit mix and ¾ cup milk with fork. Drop by spoonful into stew. Cook uncovered on low for 19 minutes. Cover and cook 10 more minutes. Makes 10–12 dumplings.

Pancakes: Beat 2 cups mix, 1 egg, and 1½ cups milk until smooth. Bake on hot griddle.

Shortcake: Mix 2 cups biscuit mix, ¾ cup cream (or ½ cup milk plus ¼ cup melted butter), and 2 tablespoons sugar with fork into a soft dough. Knead 8–10 times on floured surface. Roll to ½-inch thick. Cut with cookie cutter. Bake at 450 degrees until browned. Makes 6 servings.

Waffles: Mix 2 cups biscuit mix, 1 egg, 1²/₃ cups milk, 2 tablespoons melted butter. Cook on waffle iron.

Wheat Quick Mix

You can use this in most recipes calling for biscuit mix.

8 cups unsifted whole wheat flour
¼ cup sugar (optional)
½ cup baking powder
4 tsp. salt
1½ cups shortening (for richer mix, add 2 cups)

Mix dry ingredients together. Cut in shortening. Store in covered container up to 2 months in refrigerator.

Makes 2½ quarts.

Mix Pizza Dough

2 cups biscuit mix or wheat quick mix
½ cup water

Combine ingredients; knead one minute. Roll out and put on greased pizza pan. Add the toppings of your choice. Bake at 425 degrees for 20 minutes.

Makes one 8-inch pizza crust.

Tip! Sprinkle cornmeal on the pan to make a crispy crust.

Buttery Bread Sticks

2 cups biscuit mix or wheat quick
½ cup milk

Mix well and knead one minute. Roll out and cut into shapes or sticks. Pour melted butter in pan and put sticks in butter. Turn sticks over so the butter covers sticks. Pour more butter on top if desired. Bake at 450 degrees 12–15 minutes or until lightly brown.

Makes 6 servings.

Wheat Quick Pancakes

2 eggs
1 Tbsp. brown sugar
2 cups milk
2⅔ cups wheat quick mix

Beat eggs, brown sugar, and milk. Add wheat quick. Beat until smooth. Cook on hot griddle.

Makes 6 servings.

Wheat Quick Muffins

2 cups wheat quick mix
2 Tbsp. brown sugar
¾ cup milk
2 Tbsp. vegetable oil

Blend all ingredients. Do not overbeat. Fill greased muffin cups ¾ full. Bake at 400 degrees for 15 minutes.

Makes 12 servings.

Breakfast Sweet Bread

Bread
2 eggs, slightly beaten
¾ cup water or milk
2 cups wheat quick mix
¼ cup brown sugar
½ cup raisins

Topping
½ cup brown sugar
1–2 tsp. cinnamon
½ cup chopped nuts (optional)

Bread: Combine eggs and water or milk. Add wheat quick, brown sugar, and raisins. Pour into greased 9 x 9 pan.

Topping: Mix brown sugar, cinnamon, and nuts. Sprinkle on top of dough. Bake at 350 degrees 35–40 minutes.

Makes 8 servings.

Wheat Quick Date Bars

¼ cup soft margarine
¾ cup sugar
1 egg
1½ cups wheat quick mix
½ cup chopped nuts
1 cup chopped dates
powdered sugar

Mix margarine, sugar, and egg thoroughly. Stir in wheat quick, nuts, and dates. Bake at 350 degrees for 25 minutes in greased 8 x 8 pan. Cool 1 hour. Cut in bars and sprinkle powdered sugar on top.

Makes 9 servings.

Brownie and Chocolate Cookie Mix

4 cups flour
2 tsp. baking powder
2 tsp. salt
4 cups sugar
1½ cups cocoa
2 cups shortening

Mix dry ingredients thoroughly. Cut in shortening with pastry blender. Store in an airtight container in cool place.

Makes 2½ quarts.

Brownies

2 eggs, beaten
1 tsp. vanilla
2½ cups brownie mix
½ cup chopped nuts (optional)

Beat eggs and add vanilla. Blend in brownie mix with fork. Mix well with spoon until smooth. Stir in nuts if desired. Spread in a greased 9 x 9 pan. Bake at 350 degrees 25–30 minutes. Cool.

Makes 8 servings.

Chocolate Drop Cookies

2 eggs
¼ cup water
2¼ cups brownie mix
½ tsp. baking soda
½ cup flour
1 tsp. vanilla
pecans or walnuts, halved

Beat eggs and water in bowl with fork. Stir in brownie mix, baking soda, flour, and vanilla until blended. Drop by spoonfuls 2 inches apart on greased cookie sheets. Put a walnut or pecan half in center of each cookie. Bake at 350 degrees 10–12 minutes. Remove immediately to racks to cool.

Makes 3 dozen.

Oatmeal Mix

4 cups flour
4 cups quick-cooking oatmeal
¼ cup baking powder
1½ cups dry powdered milk
1½ cups shortening

Mix dry ingredients. Cut in shortening until well blended and crumbly. Store tightly covered in cool place. Use within a month.

Makes 10 cups.

Oatmeal Pancakes

1 cup water
1 egg
1½ cups oatmeal mix

Mix egg and water. Add oatmeal mix until smooth. Bake on hot greased griddle.

Makes 16 small pancakes.

Oatmeal Muffins

1 egg, beaten
⅔ cup water
2½ cups oatmeal mix
¼ cup raisins (optional)

Mix eggs and water. Stir in oatmeal mix and raisins just enough to moisten the mix. Fill greased muffin tin ⅔ full. Bake at 400 degrees for 20 minutes.

Makes 1 dozen.

Oatmeal Bread Sticks

½ cup butter
2 cups oatmeal mix
½ cup water

Preheat oven to 450 degrees. Melt butter in 9 x 13 pan in oven. Put oatmeal mix in bowl and add about ½ cup of water or just enough to mix ingredients together lightly with a fork. Roll out on lightly floured surface to form a rectangle. Cut in half lengthwise, and then cut each half in crosswise strips. Using fork, dip each strip in butter, coating both sides. Arrange evenly and bake at 350 degrees 12–15 minutes. Serve hot.

Makes 6 servings.

Oatmeal Mix Cookies

1 cup water
1 egg, beaten
1 tsp. vanilla
2½ cups oatmeal mix
1 tsp. cinnamon
¾ cup sugar
⅓ cup raisins

Mix water, egg, and vanilla. Add oatmeal mix, cinnamon, sugar, and raisins. Mix well. Drop by spoonfuls on greased baking sheet. Bake at 375 degrees 12–15 minutes.

Makes 2 dozen.

Muffin Mix

3 cups whole wheat flour
3 cups white flour
8 tsp. baking powder
2 tsp. salt
½ cup dry milk
1 cup shortening

Mix dry ingredients. Cut in shortening until mix is crumbly. Store in dry place.

Makes 7 cups.

Muffin Mix Muffins

2 cups muffin mix
⅓ cup water
1 egg

Mix ingredients. Fill greased muffin tins ½ full. Bake at 400 degrees for 20 minutes.

VARIATION: Fill muffin tin ¼ full. Add 1 teaspoon of jam, jelly, or fruit filling. Put more batter on top to cover the filling.

Makes 1 dozen.

Cookie Mix

8 cups sifted white flour (may use 3 cups whole wheat flour)
4½ cups sugar
4 tsp. salt
1½ tsp. baking soda
3 cups shortening

Sift dry ingredients together thoroughly. Drop shortening by spoonfuls and blend until there are no large lumps. Do not refrigerate. Keeps 6–8 weeks in your cupboard. For measuring, spoon lightly into measuring cup. Stir with fork before measuring if there are lumps.

Makes 3½ quarts.

Cocoa Raisin Drops

2 cups cookie mix
1 egg, beaten
1 Tbsp. water
¼ cup sugar
1 tsp. vanilla
1 baking chocolate square, melted
½ cup raisin

Blend cookie mix with egg and water. Blend in sugar, vanilla, and chocolate. Add raisins. Drop on cookie sheet. Bake at 350 degrees 10–12 minutes. Cool on rack.

Makes 1 dozen.

Coconut Macaroons

1 egg
1 Tbsp. milk
1½ tsp. vanilla or almond flavoring
2 cups cookie mix
2 cups coconut

Mix egg, milk, and flavoring. Blend in cookie mix. Add coconut until evenly mixed. Drop on cookie sheet. Bake at 350 degrees 15–17 minutes or until golden brown. Cool before serving.

Makes 2 dozen.

Date Clusters

1½ tsp. vanilla
1 egg
3 cups cookie mix
½ cup brown sugar
½ cup chopped nuts
1 cup chopped dates

Mix vanilla, egg, and cookie mix until smooth and fluffy. Stir in sugar, nuts, and dates until evenly blended. Drop on greased cookie sheet with spoon. Bake at 375 degrees 10–12 minutes or until lightly brown. Remove immediately from pan.

Makes 2 dozen.

Quick Pudding Mix

1½ cups sugar
1½ cups cornstarch
1 tsp. salt
14 cups dry milk powder

Mix all ingredients well. Store in airtight container. Keep on pantry shelf.

To use: Heat 2½ cups water. Gradually stir in 1½ cups mix into saucepan. Bring to a boil on low heat. Stir constantly until thick.

Makes 6-8 servings, or will fill one 8-inch pie shell.

VARIATIONS (ADD THE FOLLOWING WHILE BOILING)

Chocolate: Add 2 tablespoons chocolate syrup.

Fruit and Nuts: Add ½ cup crushed pineapple, apricots, shredded coconut, or nuts. Garnish with chocolate cookie crumbs and top with whipped cream. Brown at 400 degrees.

Peppermint: Add ½ cup crushed peppermint candy.

Vanilla: Add ½ teaspoon vanilla and 1 teaspoon butter.

DELUXE VARIATIONS

Banana Cream Pie: Slice 3–4 bananas in baked pie shell. Cover with vanilla pudding and whipped cream.

Coconut Cream Pie: Double vanilla pudding recipe; add 1 cup coconut. Fill pie shell and top with whipped cream.

Parfait: Spoon alternating layers of vanilla pudding, thickened fruit, berries, and chocolate pudding in parfait glasses.

Parfait Pie: When pudding is cool, layer like parfait dessert as above. Put in baked pie shell and top with whipped cream.

Vanilla Pudding: Mix 1 cup plus 3 tablespoons pudding mix, 3 drops of yellow food coloring, and 1 small egg (optional). Set aside. Bring 1¼ cups of water to a boil. Add pudding mixture. Stir on medium heat until mixture bubbles about 15 minutes. Remove. Stir in 2 tablespoons butter and 1 teaspoon vanilla. Garnish with sliced peaches, other fruit, or chocolate sauce, if desired. Makes 4 servings.

Hot Cocoa Mix

8 qts. dry milk powder
2 cups cocoa
2–3 cups powdered sugar
½ tsp. salt

Mix all ingredients and store tightly closed container. To serve, use 2–3 tablespoons cocoa mix per cup of hot water.

Beef Gravy Mix

1½ cups dry milk powder
¾ cup white flour
2 Tbsp. beef bouillon granules
3–4 tsp. pepper
½ cup butter

Mix dry ingredients. Cut in butter until mixture is like cornmeal. Store in tightly covered container in the refrigerator.

Makes 2½ cups.

To use: Blend in saucepan, 1 cup cold water, ½ cup beef gravy mix, and a few drops beef broth or soy sauce. Stir until mixture is thick and bubbly. Cook 1 minute; continue to stir.

Soup Mix

1 (14-oz) pkg. alphabet macaroni
1 (14-oz.) pkg. dry green split peas
1½ cups white or brown rice or cracked wheat
1 (12-oz.) pkg. instant pearl barley

Tip! Add meat bones for flavoring with the 2 quarts of water.

Mix well together. Store tightly covered.

To use: In large pot, mix 2 quarts water, vegetable or beef stock, 1⅓ cups soup mix, 1 tablespoon plus 1 teaspoon salt, and 2 bouillon cubes (optional). Cover, bring to a boil, turn heat to low, and simmer 1 hour. Add 2 diced carrots, 1 stalk chopped celery, ¼ head of chopped cabbage, ½–1 chopped onion, and 2 (8-oz.) cans tomato sauce. Simmer until vegetables are tender.

Makes 8 servings.

Seasoning Mix

Use this for chicken, fish, or pork.

3 cups fine dry bread crumbs (or mix with half wheat germ)
3 Tbsp. onion powder
1 Tbsp. salt
2 tsp. poultry seasoning
½ tsp. garlic powder
¾ tsp. paprika
¾ tsp. dried thyme, crushed
⅛ tsp. cayenne

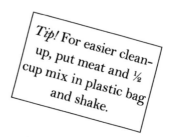

Tip! For easier clean-up, put meat and ½ cup mix in plastic bag and shake.

Mix and store in tightly covered quart jar.

To use: Dip pieces of meat in milk and then in seasoning. Bake or fry according to recipe.

Makes 1 quart.

Seasoning Mix Variation

Use this for chicken, fish, or pork.

4 cups dried bread crumbs
½ cup flour
1 Tbsp. paprika
4 tsp. salt
4 tsp. sugar
4 tsp. onion powder
1 tsp. garlic powder
½ cup shortening

Mix dry ingredients and cut in shortening. Store in covered jar.

To use: Dip pieces in milk and then in seasoning or shake seasoning in bag with meat. Bake or fry according to recipe.

Makes 1 quart.

Spanish Rice Mix

4 cups uncooked rice
4 tsp. parsley flakes
½ cup green bell pepper flakes
4 tsp. salt
1 tsp. dried basil

Mix well. Store in tightly closed container.

Makes 8 cups.

To use: Bring 1 cup plus 2 tablespoons rice mix, 1 tablespoon butter, and 2 cups water to boil in heavy saucepan. Cover tightly and cook over low heat for 15 minutes or until liquid is absorbed.

Makes 4–6 servings.

Beef Jerky

1 beef flank steak
½ cup soy sauce
½ tsp. garlic salt
¼ tsp. lemon pepper

Trim all visible fat from beef. Cut lengthwise with grain into long thin strips, no more than ¼-inch thick. (If steak is slightly frozen it will slice easier.) Combine soy sauce and seasonings. Pour over beef strips and toss until meat is well coated. Place a wire rack on a baking sheet. Arrange strips on rack to touch but not overlap. Arrange in center of oven no closer than four inches from top or bottom. Bake at 150 degrees 10–12 hours or until very dry. Store at room temperature in an airtight container.

If all fat has been removed, beef jerky will keep many years. If jerky is crisp, the oven was too hot. If jerky is not quite dry enough, white specks may appear after a few days. Keeps best in refrigerator.

Egg Substitute

This is for baking only.

Combine 1 teaspoon unflavored gelatin with 3 tablespoons cold water and 2 tablespoons plus 1 teaspoon boiling water.

Substitutes 1 egg.

Cinnamon-Sugar Blend

2 Tbsp. sugar
½ tsp. cinnamon

Mix. Store in a salt or pepper shaker. Use on toast, cereal, and so forth.

Powdered Sugar Substitute

1½ Tbsp. cornstarch
1 lb. granulated sugar

Blend together at highest speed until very fine.

Brown Sugar Substitute

2 cups granulated sugar
1 Tbsp. blackstrap molasses

Tip! If it is hard, you used too much molasses. Just add more granulated sugar.

Put in bowl and mix with fork or rub together with hands.

Diet Margarine

Slowly warm 1 cup margarine on lowest heat on stove until nearly melted. Remove from heat. Stir to break up remaining pieces. Add ½ cup milk. Beat milk into melted margarine until thoroughly blended and creamy in texture. For a thicker consistency, add dry milk powder. The volume will nearly double. Store in refrigerator. Makes 1¾ cups.

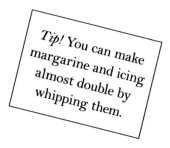

Tip! You can make margarine and icing almost double by whipping them.

Condensed Milk Substitute

Mix ¼ cup hot water, 1 cup powdered milk, and 1 cup sugar in blender. For more flavor, add ¼ cup butter. Can be stored in refrigerator or even frozen.

Buttermilk Substitute

Mix 1 cup water, ⅓ cup milk powder, and 1 tablespoon vinegar or lemon juice.

Homemade Buttermilk

Mix 3¾ cups water and 1⅓ cups instant milk powder in large bowl. (Use blender if non-instant dry milk is used.) Stir in ½ cup fresh buttermilk. Cover with waxed paper and clean towel. Let stand in a warm room until curdled (usually overnight). Stir until smooth. Store in the refrigerator. Makes approximately 1 quart. You can save ½ cup of this buttermilk to make your next quart.

Homemade Cottage Cheese

Mix 7½ cups water and 2⅔ cups instant nonfat dry milk (or 2⅓ cups non-instant dry milk) in large bowl. (Use blender if non-instant dry milk is used.) Stir in 1 cup buttermilk. Cover with waxed paper or clean towel. Let stand in warm room until curdled (usually overnight). Pour into large, heavy saucepan. Cook over low heat for 1 hour or until curd is firm enough to hold its shape when pressed gently between the fingers. Pour mixture into strainer lined with cheesecloth. Rinse with cold water. Put cheese in bowl. Mix gently with ½ teaspoon salt. For moister cottage cheese, add ½ cup homemade buttermilk or ½ cup liquid milk. Cover and chill before serving. Store in refrigerator.

Makes 2 cups.

Yogurt

8 cups whole milk
1 container plain yogurt (no additives)

Scald milk. Let cool to lukewarm or until you can hold your little finger in milk to the count of 10. In a small bowl, mix plain yogurt until smooth. Add milk and stir. Make sure yogurt culture is evenly distributed. Cover and wrap in thick towel. Do not disturb. Keep in warm place for at least ten hours. It should be thick before refrigerating. It will also thicken in the fridge. As you use yogurt, parts of it will get thin and watery. This part can be used for yogurt spread (recipe below).

Tip! The liquid can be used in making bread.

Yogurt Spread

Pour yogurt in strainer lined with a coffee filter. Let liquid strain out for several hours or overnight. Use the thickened yogurt in the coffee filter as a spread.

Whipped Topping

½ cup dry powdered milk
⅓ cup cold water
1 Tbsp. lemon juice
3 Tbsp. sugar
2 tsp. vanilla

Chill bowl and beater in the refrigerator. Beat powdered milk and water together until it starts to thicken. Add lemon juice and beat until it forms soft peaks. Add sugar and vanilla and beat a few more minutes.

Creme Fraiche

This is used in many French recipes.

1 pint sour cream
1 Tbsp. lemon juice or vinegar
1 Tbsp. sugar (optional)

Mix together and let sit on the counter overnight or about 12 hours. Add sugar if desired.

Homemade Household Products

All-Purpose Cleaner

1 tsp. borax
2 Tbsp. lemon juice
1 Tbsp. flour with a few drops water
1 cup hot water

Combine ingredients in a pint-sized spray bottle. Shake until dry ingredients are dissolved.

Window Cleaner

These will clean and cut grease and dirt.

¼ cup plain ammonia
4 cups water

or

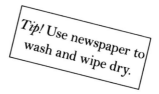

Tip! Use newspaper to wash and wipe dry.

2 Tbsp. nonsudsy ammonia
2 cups rubbing alcohol
1 gallon water (in jug)

Mix in container with lid. Label container.

Stove and Tub Cleaner

vinegar
cream of tartar

Make a paste using equal parts of vinegar and cream of tartar. Use with a scouring pad or sponge. Mix with water to clean tub or stove.

Tub and Tile Cleaner

1 cup baking soda
1 cup ammonia
1 cup white vinegar
4 cups warm water

Mix all ingredients together in a spray bottle. Apply directly to tile. Wipe off with damp sponge.

Toilet Cleaner

1 cup borax (found in drug store)
½ cup white vinegar

Flush the toilet to wet the sides. Sprinkle borax along insides of bowl. Drizzle vinegar over borax and leave overnight. Scrub with a toilet brush and flush.

WARNING: Borax is poisonous! Avoid contact or ingestion for humans and animals.

Toilet Cleaner Variation

8 cups water
1 cup hydrogen peroxide
1 Tbsp. ammonia

Put ingredients in spray bottle and spray insides of toilet bowl. Let sit 30 minutes or more. Flush and scrub off.

This mix will fit into a duck-shaped toilet cleaner bottle: 4 cups water, ¼ cup hydrogen peroxide, and 1 teaspoon ammonia.

Laundry Bleach

1 cup hydrogen peroxide

Add to a load of whites instead of bleach to whiten a load of laundry. Pour hydrogen peroxide directly on a soiled spot. Let it sit for a minute, then rub and rinse with cold water. Repeat if necessary.

Stain Remover

1–3 Tbsp. hydrogen peroxide
1–3 Tbsp. baking soda

Pour hydrogen peroxide on stain and sprinkle generously with baking soda. Rub it in. Let it sit 1–24 hours. Wash as usual.

WARNING: You may want to test stain remover on a place where it's not seen to be sure it doesn't bleach the material.

Baby Wipes

3 cups water
2 Tbsp. baby oil
2 Tbsp. baby shampoo
½ roll thick paper towels

Cut the paper towel roll in half. Remove the center core so you can pull paper towel from the middle. Use a tightly covered plastic container that the towels fit into. Make a slit in the top to pull the paper towel through. Put all the liquid in the plastic container and stir. Put in half the paper towel roll. Pull the paper towel from middle and push it through the slit in lid. Fit lid tightly on container and tip upside down until paper towels absorb moisture. You should be able to pull one at a time and have each one moist as you use it.

Toothbrush Cleaner

¼ cup hydrogen peroxide

Soak your toothbrushes in hydrogen peroxide to prevent germ buildup. Change the hydrogen peroxide every few days or once a week. This also helps prevent colds and germs from spreading in families.

Teeth Whitener

This is a great scrub and teeth whitener.

baking soda
hydrogen peroxide

Make a paste of baking soda and drops of hydrogen peroxide in palm of your hand. Dip toothbrush in paste and brush.

Liquid Deodorant

1 Tbsp. powdered alum
1½ cups water
1 Tbsp. rubbing alcohol

Pour in plastic spray bottle. You can scent this deodorant with your favorite cologne or perfume instead of water. Shake before each use.

Cream Deodorant

1 tsp. petroleum jelly
1 tsp. talcum powder
1 tsp. baking soda

Mix these and place in the top of a double boiler. Heat and stir constantly until smooth. Scrape the mixture into a clean jar and keep covered. Apply with cosmetic pad or fingers.

Deodorant Powder

This will absorb odor for up to 6 hours.

½ cup baking soda
¼ cup medicated powder

Mix together and pour the powder into a salt or pepper shaker. Sprinkle liberally.

Cough Suppressant

Sip liquid for cough.

4 tsp. ginger
1 onion, finely chopped
1½ cups sugar
6 cups water

Simmer all ingredients at least 30 minutes. Strain liquid through a coffee filter.

NOTE: This is high in sugar and therefore not advisable for diabetics or others on sugar-free diets.

Mustard Plaster for Congestion

This is a rub for the chest.

3 Tbsp. dry mustard
1 Tbsp. flour
a few drops water

Combine to make a paste. Place thin cloth on chest and spread mixture on cloth. As it dries it will warm the chest and loosen the cough.

WARNING: Not for consumption.

Flea and Tick Spray

1 Tbsp. dried rosemary
1 Tbsp. dried fennel
1 Tbsp. dried eucalyptus (found in health food stores)
1 cup water

Mix all ingredients. Store in small spray bottle.

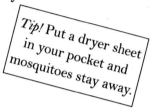

Tip! Put a dryer sheet in your pocket and mosquitoes stay away.

Roach and Insect Repellent

¼ cup shortening
¼ cup sugar
½ cup onion, finely chopped
½ cup flour
1 cup boric acid (found in drug store)
water

Mix ingredients in a gallon-sized ziplock plastic bag. Add enough water to form a soft dough. Place a small marble-size ball in bottle caps where insects live or where you have seen unwanted insects. Be sure to clean measuring cups before using again.

WARNING: Boric acid is poisonous! Avoid contact or ingestion for humans and animals.

Ant Killer

Place small amount of cornmeal where ants appear. They will take it to their nest. Ants can't digest cornmeal and will die.

Index

About the Author

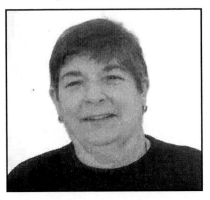

Anne Casbeer is the oldest of four siblings. She spent most of her young life in the New England states of Massachusetts and New Hampshire. She graduated from Brigham Young University with a B.S. in food and nutrition. As an officer in the army she interned at Walter Reed General Hospital in nutrition and became a registered dietitian. She worked as a registered dietitian in the army and was honorably discharged as a first lieutenant. She then worked as a dietitian and managed a bakery.